Storytelling Encounters as Medical Education

This innovative volume provides fresh perspectives on how medical students and patients construct identities in relation to each other, using stories of their clinical encounters. It explores how paying attention to medical students' and patients' stories in clinical teaching encounters can encourage empathy and the formation of professional identities that embody desirable values such as integrity and respect.

Written by an experienced clinician and based on original, rigorous research combining ethnography and dialogic narrative analysis, *Storytelling Encounters as Medical Education: Crafting Relational Identity* includes patient stories alongside those of students and clinical teachers.

This is an important contribution for all those interested in medical education, narrative medicine, person-centred care and identity formation in healthcare. It will also be of value to scholars in a range of other disciplines, who are using a dialogic approach.

Sally G. Warmington is an honorary fellow at the Melbourne School of Population and Global Health, University of Melbourne, Australia and a retired medical doctor. Her research interests include storytelling and relational identity, relationships and ethics in the clinical encounter, and patient experiences of participation in medical education.

Routledge Advances in the Medical Humanities

For more information about this series visit: www.routledge.com/Routledge-Advances-in-the-Medical-Humanities/book-series/RAMH

Storytelling Encounters as Medical Education
Crafting Relational Identity

Sally G. Warmington

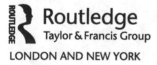

Routledge
Taylor & Francis Group

LONDON AND NEW YORK

First published 2020 by Routledge

2 Park Square, Milton Park, Abingdon, Oxon OX14 4RN
605 Third Avenue, New York, NY 10017

Routledge is an imprint of the Taylor & Francis Group, an informa business

First issued in paperback 2021

Publisher's Note

The publisher has gone to great lengths to ensure the quality of this reprint but points out that some imperfections in the original copies may be apparent.

British Library Cataloguing-in-Publication Data
A catalogue record for this book is available from the British Library

Library of Congress Cataloging-in-Publication Data
A catalog record has been requested for this book

ISBN: 978-0-367-32206-9 (hbk)
ISBN: 978-1-03-217700-7 (pbk)
DOI: 10.4324/9780429317262

Typeset in Times New Roman
by Wearset Ltd, Boldon, Tyne and Wear

Dedicated to
Mikhail Mikhailovich Bakhtin
1895–1975

Contents

Figures

Acknowledgements

This book is adapted from the ethnographic text of my doctoral dissertation, completed in 2013 at the Melbourne School of Population and Global Health at the University of Melbourne, Australia, where I continue as an honorary fellow. I acknowledge that the University is situated on the land of the Wurundjeri people of the Kulin nation, and I pay my respect to their elders – past, present and emerging.

Some of the material in Chapter 6 has been adapted with permission from Springer Nature, previously published in the journal *Advances in Health Sciences Education* (2016) as 'Medical student stories of participation in patient care-related activities: the construction of relational identity', by Sally Warmington and Geoff McColl.

Many people have contributed to this book or influenced its development and I am thankful to them all, although I can only name some of them here. Firstly, I want to acknowledge my research participants: the students, patients and clinical teachers who generously shared their stories and allowed me to witness their clinical encounters.

I am deeply grateful for the expertise, interest and commitment of my PhD supervisors, Marilys Guillemin, Geoff McColl and Richard Chenhall. Throughout my candidature, they supported my development as a scholar and engaged with my ongoing struggles. The diversity of their backgrounds prompted me to draw on literature from many disciplines. During that time, I also received generous support and advice from Lynn Gillam, Robyn Woodward-Kron, Celia Thompson, Michelle Leech and many other colleagues.

It has been a great source of encouragement when scholars whose ideas have informed and inspired me – notably Lynn Monrouxe, Alan Bleakley and Arthur Frank – have responded positively to my work. I offer my sincere thanks to those who have generously read and responded to this manuscript: Jenny Barrett, Alan Bleakley, Peter Cantillon, Richard Chenhall, Mahtab Janfada, May-Lill Johansen, Geoff McColl, Lynn Monrouxe and Hamish Wilson.

The graphics that enhance this book were created by design and data visualisation consultant Alana Pirrone, through our close collaboration and her enthusiastic engagement with the manuscript.

My thanks to Ruth Anderson and the editorial team at Routledge, whose prompt, helpful advice has made preparing my book for publication a very positive experience.

I am deeply grateful to Oliver Larkin for giving me the opportunity to experience at first hand the healing power of dialogue.

Sincere thanks to my family for their support, especially my late mother Rae who taught me to love reading, and my father Stuart, who embodies the joy of creativity. To my daughters Cathy Vanderzeil and Angie Vanderzeil: my life and work are enriched by your support, encouragement, kindness and love.

1   Storytelling matters

People often say to me, 'Oh, Daniel, you always get great stories out of the patients – how come?' So, when I'm handing over, I'll say: 'Oh this is so and so, and actually, he fought in Papua New Guinea and was on the Kokoda Trail', or: 'She went and worked up in the Northern Territory', or something like that. By telling a story about them, it makes them human again. I find that helps other doctors, other staff, to connect with that person as a real person, and not as a disease.

Daniel, emergency physician and clinical teacher

Background

Throughout my 35 years in medical practice, I have been both intrigued and troubled by the relationships between doctors and patients. This book, based on my own research, takes a close look at encounters between hospital patients and medical students in their first clinical year. As newcomers to the hospital, medical students offer novel perspectives on the clinical encounters that happen there. My research also explores patients' experiences of interacting with students and clinical teachers. Patient stories about being involved in clinical teaching have received limited attention in the literature, but offer important insights. The voices of clinical teachers are also relevant because they are key players in many interactions between students and patients.

In this book I explore identity in medical education as a dynamic, relational phenomenon, offering a fresh perspective informed by social theory and anthropological research. One of the ways people construct and perform identities in everyday life is through interactive storytelling. Medical educators appreciate that understanding and supporting the development of learners' professional identity is as important as advancing their knowledge and skills (Goldie, 2012; Cruess, Cruess, Boudreau, Snell, & Steinert, 2014; Monrouxe, 2010). It is less widely recognised that identity construction is an integral part of *all* clinical teaching and learning.

Narrative, storytelling and identity

Language plays a central role in identity construction and performance, although non-verbal means also contribute. The clothes we wear and the way we physically interact with others, for example, can communicate a great deal about who we are (Iedema & Caldas-Coulthard, 2008, p. 6). In this book, my focus is mainly on the use of language, both because of my interest in story-telling and because my data consists mainly of verbal records of interviews and other encounters. The terms *narrative* and *story* sometimes convey different meanings, although I often use them interchangeably in this book as nouns, while I also use *narrative* as an adjective. One distinction I make is that some narratives arise and circulate as part of the cultures with which people identify. These shared narratives are a resource we draw upon to construct our own personal stories (Frank, 2010).

Researchers in the human sciences have a strong interest in stories, recognising them as objects for study in their own right, and not merely as vehicles for the transmission of data (Garro & Mattingly, 2000; Bleakley, 2005). An appreciation of the power of storytelling can be linked in the Western world to an enduring fascination with language, autobiography and the self (Reissman, 2008). Storytelling is a way of bringing together the worlds of action and consciousness, and making meaning from experience (Garro & Mattingly, 2000). Stories can be understood as actors in the social world because they can make things happen by influencing those who hear them (Frank, 2010).

A story is an account with certain characteristics, including a description of events in which something happens as a result of a previous event. In a fully developed story, a pattern or *narrative arc* is usually followed: the scene is set, an unexpected or troubling event occurs, and suspense develops as to how it will be resolved. After the resolution, the narrator offers an evaluation of characters and events (Frank, 2010). There is a consequential relationship between events in even the simplest story. Most of the stories in this book were produced through interactive talk. In these situations, a story may be quite short and lack some of these elements (Gubrium & Holstein, 2009).

Narrators always select and organise their story's component parts to suit their intended audiences. In other words, a story is always *recipient-designed*, whether this is done deliberately or not (Frank, 2010; Reissman, 2008). The way we transcribe recordings of interviews and other interactions can influence the stories that emerge from that data. For this project, interactions were transcribed word for word as far as possible, noting the tone or volume of a speaker's voice, any hesitation or laughter and including my contributions as the interviewer. This approach allows a deeper understanding of the context in which a story was told and provides access to the small story fragments that populate people's conversations (Sools, 2013).

Stories serve many purposes. Autobiographical stories can help us understand the past, as lived experiences are given form and evaluated by narrators, often in collaboration with others. This is a key process in psychotherapy and in many research settings. Stories can also shape the future, because the insights gained from telling or listening to a story can influence people's actions (Garro & Mattingly, 2000). Crucially for this project, they convey something about the character or identity of the narrator and characters in the story, and often persuade us to interpret events from the narrator's perspective (Frank, 2010).

Narrative and identity are linked in the concept of *master narratives*: stories told and authorised by powerful or higher status groups within a society (Nelson, 2001). Master narratives identify members of less powerful or lower status social groups in particular ways. The persistence of these stories can constrain the identities that those depicted in them are able to construct for themselves, and consequently the ways in which they can act in the world. However, they may construct *counter-stories*, resisting the identities imposed upon them by those in more powerful positions. This illustrates how the rhetorical or persuasive functions of a story can be used for political as well as social ends (Garro & Mattingly, 2000; Nelson, 2001).

While I highlight the important relationship between storytelling and identity, I acknowledge the argument that some people do not perceive their lives as having a narrative quality. Strawson (2004) argues that it is possible to flourish and live an ethically good life without thinking narratively. This argument seems to be based on the idea of narrative as the story of a person's life, with a recognisable narrative structure. In contrast, I am interested in the small story fragments from everyday human interactions. These may be considered autobiographical in that they contain stories from or about the narrator's life, but they need not be integrated into a coherent whole. Besides, not all stories are well-structured – indeed, some illness narratives have a chaotic quality, and their lack of coherence can express their narrators' bewildering experience more eloquently than the words from which they are composed (Middlebrook, 1996; Rimmon-Kenan, 2002; De Peuter, 1998).

During my fieldwork I often discussed with students their encounters with patients. Many students wondered why their attempts to elicit the history of a patient's illness often resulted in long, rambling stories. When I examined these stories closely, I realised that they accomplish much more than just the transmission of facts. Whenever someone tells a story, they also convey something about who they are in relation to others. This *identity work* takes place whenever people interact with each other. In a teaching hospital, this can include patients, doctors, nurses, allied health professionals, family members and housekeeping staff as well as students. In this book, I focus on encounters between medical students and patients, which often involve doctors as well in a teaching or supervisory capacity.

Aims

I have several aims in writing this book. The first is to show how students and patients use interactive storytelling to construct identities in relation to each other. Identity work is an integral part of all learning interactions. When clinical teachers recognise that identity work is taking place, they can encourage learners to reflect about it. Gaining insight into the struggles associated with identity formation may help educators to support medical students and doctors-in-training through times of conflict or distress (Dyrbye, Thomas, & Shanafelt, 2005; Monrouxe, 2010).

Secondly, I want to demonstrate why paying attention to patients' stories in medical education is important, even when they seem irrelevant to the presenting problem. These stories may offer insights into patients' experiences of participating in clinical teaching, which can be positive, negative or mixed. Clinical teachers who appreciate this are better placed to reduce the likelihood of discomfort or harm to patients and maximise the potential for benefit (Chretien, Goldman, Craven, & Faselis, 2010; Nair, Coughlan, & Hensley, 1997; Rice, 2008). In this book, I use stories to explore the inter-relationship between identity, power dynamics and ethics in clinical teaching and learning interactions. This offers insights into how patients are recruited for clinical teaching, and how some common practices can compromise the validity of their consent to participate.

Finally, I will show how appreciating the importance of storytelling can humanise the practice of clinical teaching and care. A patient becomes a unique individual when they are given space to tell stories about their life, and again when these self-identifying stories are shared with other people. Without them, a person can be perceived as just another case of some condition. Storytelling opens a window into patients' lives and helps students and clinicians relate to them with empathy and compassion.

Outline of theory and methods

A detailed explanation of my research methods and supporting theory can be found in Chapter 2. This brief outline shows how my research relates to the published work discussed later in this chapter. The theoretical foundation for the study on which this book is based is the work of Mikhail Bakhtin, a Russian theorist and literary critic who proposed that human relations are best understood as a *dialogue* (Gardiner & Bell, 1998). By this he meant that people construct *selves* – analogous to identities – in relation to the people they interact with, and that this process involves a creative struggle (Holquist, 2002). Bakhtin's ideas influenced social theorist and psychoanalyst Julia Kristeva, who proposed the idea of the self as dynamic and constantly changing (Guberman, 1996). Like Bakhtin, Kristeva highlights negotiation and struggle as essential to identity construction.

I used an ethnographic approach to study medical student and patient encounters in a large metropolitan teaching hospital in Australia. I was interested in how medical students and patients experience and interpret their interactions with each other in a teaching hospital. Ethnographic researchers spend extended periods of time, often months or years, engaged in the practice of *fieldwork*. This involves immersion in the everyday life of a cultural group, collecting stories through observations and interactions, including interviews and informal conversations.

After obtaining approval from the relevant ethics committees, I recruited three groups of participants: students in their first clinical year, patients and clinical teachers. I gathered stories from observations of clinical teaching interactions and undertook in-depth, semi-structured interviews. After repeated reading of the transcribed data and listening to the audio recordings, I constructed tables and charts highlighting important stories and drawing links between them. I observed emerging themes and connections, and selected stories for deeper analysis that were most salient to my research focus, as well as those that were surprising or especially moving.

I analysed these stories using a process called *dialogic narrative analysis*, focusing on how a story was produced and performed within a particular context (Gubrium & Holstein, 2009; Reissman, 2008). I incorporated elements of critical discourse analysis, enabling meanings to emerge from the way a story was told as well as its content. This involved looking closely at how language was used within a story to convey context-specific meanings. I identified multiple voices used by a single narrator and juxtaposed stories told by different narrators, placing them *in dialogue* with each other. Finally, I considered what had been accomplished by telling a given story in a particular context (Frank, 2010).

Crafting relational identity

Daniel's story

To explain what I mean when I describe identity as *relational*, let's take a closer look at the story that opens this chapter. Daniel was a clinical teacher who participated in my research. Towards the end of our interview, I mentioned my interest in storytelling, and he offered this tale about the importance of stories in his own clinical practice as an emergency physician.

> People often say to me, 'Oh, Daniel, you always get great stories out of the patients – how come?' So, when I'm handing over, I'll say: 'Oh this is so and so, and actually, he fought in Papua New Guinea and was on the Kokoda Trail', or: 'She went and worked up in the Northern Territory', or something like that. By telling a story about them, it makes them human again. I find that helps other doctors, other staff, to connect with that person as a real person, and not as a disease.

Daniel claims that the act of storytelling does important work for patients: 'it makes them human again'. He makes two important points here: that patients' humanity is somehow in need of restoration; and that we can make a connection with a patient through stories about their life. However, when we examine his story more closely, it becomes clear that he is also telling us about himself. Another way of saying this is that he is doing *identity work*, which is an integral part of everyday storytelling interactions and often takes place without the narrator being aware of it.

One way that people accomplish this is by using multiple voices in the telling of the story, producing a *multi-vocal narrative*, of which this short excerpt is an excellent example. Daniel speaks with three voices: that of another staff member, his own voice as a character in the story and his own voice as the narrator. He

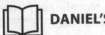

DANIEL'S STORY - A MULTI-VOCAL NARRATIVE

Voice of unnamed staff member

"Oh, Daniel, you always get great stories out of the patients – how come?"

Voice of Daniel as a character in the story

"Oh, this is so and so, and actually, he fought in Papua New Guinea and was on the Kokoda Trail", or: "She went and worked up in the Northern Territory."

Voice of Daniel as narrator

By telling a story about them, it makes them human again. I find that helps other doctors, other staff, to connect with that person as a real person, and not as a disease.

Figure 1.1 Daniel's story: a multi-vocal narrative.

conveys his assessment of the characters by *speaking through* their words, giving us the impression that they are speaking directly to us. This technique is called *ventriloquation* because the narrator's voice is like that of a ventriloquist who creates the illusion that their mannequin is speaking. The first voice we hear is that of an unnamed staff member, who asks:

'Oh, Daniel, you always get great stories out of the patients – how come?'

Daniel then speaks with his own voice as a character in the story he is telling:

'Oh, this is so and so, and actually, he fought in Papua New Guinea and was on the Kokoda Trail', or: 'She went and worked up in the Northern Territory'.

Finally, he speaks with his own voice as narrator, giving a rationale for this practice:

By telling a story about them, it makes them human again. I find that helps other doctors, other staff, to connect with that person as a real person, and not as a disease.

Through the use and juxtaposition of these three voices, Daniel constructs and performs his identity in relation to others. He characterises himself and the other staff in certain ways, juxtaposes these characters and adopts a position in relation to them. In this story, he identifies himself as a more humane, compassionate doctor than his colleagues. Because it is told in the context of the interview, he also identifies himself in relation to me, as a colleague with shared values in relation to storytelling and the pursuit of meaningful clinical relationships.

This brief analysis shows how identity is constructed relationally through storytelling in everyday interactions. I provide more details in the next chapter about the theory and practical steps used to produce the analysis. Throughout this book, I use a similar approach to analyse stories told by students, patients and clinical teachers during their interactions with each other or in research interviews. This novel approach to studying identity in medical education has led to a number of original findings, with important implications for clinical teaching and patient care.

Social and cultural research on identity

Researchers have employed a variety of theories and methods to study identity in medical education (Monrouxe & Rees, 2015; Bleakley, Bligh, & Browne, 2011; Dornan, Pearson, Carson, Helmich, & Bundy, 2015; Goldie, 2012). In this review, I focus on social science and humanities research, especially from anthropology, social psychology, sociolinguistics and the medical humanities. Researchers in these disciplines view identity as a social phenomenon that emerges when people interact with each other. I will begin by introducing contemporary social and cultural ideas about the nature of identity and its construction, then discuss narrative approaches to identity research in medical education.

A dynamic and relational phenomenon

Identity used to be thought of as relatively stable in adult life but is now understood as an active and ongoing process, linking our lived experience and the social systems of practices, values and beliefs in which we live and work. One way in which people construct identities is through a narrative device known as *interactional positioning* (Wortham, 2000). This refers to storytellers' practice of conveying something about their own character or identity by characterising others in certain ways and locating themselves socially in relation to those others. As we saw in Daniel's story, narrators position themselves in relation to audiences, conversation partners and characters in their stories, including their own present and former selves. They can also position themselves in relation to ideologies, practices and power structures, either aligning themselves with or distancing themselves from them (De Fina, Schiffrin, & Bamberg, 2006). Studies of identity formation in school classrooms have highlighted the fact that academic learning, identity formation and the power dynamics of learning interactions are inextricably linked (Wortham, 2006).

The idea that identities are constructed and performed in the moment, but also form a more enduring aspect of an individual, presents us with a paradox. The notion of *timescales* has been proposed as a way to resolve this (Lemke,

2008). We can think about identities as developing over a spectrum of time-scales, ranging from a single interaction to many interactions over a longer period of time. The link between longer and shorter-term identities can be understood in terms of *recurrence*. Our identities become more stable and enduring because of recurring contact with people with whom we have relationships, objects with a particular meaning and situations we recognise as requiring particular responses. In this book, I focus on the ways we construct and perform identity in the moment. The methods I used to gather, transcribe and analyse the stories allowed a close examination of identity work in a short timescale. Investigating the relationship between short-term and longer-term identities in medical education could be considered as a future project.

The materiality and endurance of our physical bodies, with sensory memories, embodied habits, perceptions, skills and needs, are critical to the continuity of our identities. Because these conditions can alter over time, identities are also subject to change, being *fluid* to the extent that we can choose to identify ourselves in some ways and not in others. However, the choices available to any individual are constrained by a number of factors including previous experiences, the current context and the social groups that person identifies with (Lemke, 2008).

From the time we first become aware that we are separate beings, our desires and fears are related to the needs and vulnerabilities of our bodies. The use of physical and emotional pain in the socialisation of children, for example by physical punishment or the replacement of positive regard by disapproval, is one means by which cultures come to shape our identities. We are subjected to social pressures to perform particular identities from early childhood and throughout adult life: 'to conform and to dissemble' (Lemke, 2008, p. 27).

Because our values and beliefs about who we are in relation to others are associated with fears and desires, they can have a powerful influence on our identities and are useful considerations for a dialogic narrative analysis. Although they may not be articulated, inferences can be drawn about the fears and desires expressed through a story, and how they contribute to the narrator's identity (Frank, 2010). For example, several stories in this book explore the tension for students between prioritising a patient's needs and performing as successful members of the medical community. The fear of looking foolish and the desire to appear proficient emerge as powerful motivating factors.

The importance of power dynamics in the construction of identity has been studied in relation to school classroom learning (Wortham, 2006, 2008) and medical education (Donetto, 2012; Holmes, Jenks, & Stonington, 2011; Rees, Ajjawi, & Monrouxe, 2013). Medical students are not passively socialised, but instead, are 'active subjects who make choices, resist subjugation, incorporate power differentials, and actively craft themselves internally' as they learn (Holmes et al., 2011, p. 109). This book highlights how the identities of students and patients are shaped as they resist or submit to cultural expectations.

Traditionally, theories of learning and identity have considered identity construction separately from the acquisition of knowledge and skills. Situated learning theory highlights how people learn through increasing levels of participation in occupational groups, or *communities of practice* (Lave & Wenger, 1991; Wenger, 1998). From this perspective, identity construction is an integral part of learning and is influenced by the context in which it takes place. However, this theory pays limited attention to the way people actively position themselves in relation to others; it does not consider that identities are multiple, nor does it address factors that expand or limit people's potential identities.

The sociocultural approach to identity construction addresses some of the limitations of situated learning theory (Vågan, 2011). According to this perspective, identities emerge as people position themselves as particular kinds of people within certain social contexts. It integrates interactional positioning (Wortham, 2000, 2001) and *figured worlds* theory (Dornan et al., 2015; Vågan, 2011). A figured world is a social context in which particular characters are identified and recognised; for example, the world of romantic love in college students, or the world of becoming a doctor in medical school (Vågan, 2011). We characterise our identities in a figured world by positioning ourselves in relation to simplified versions of characters, objects, actions and consequences.

The construction of meaning and identities can be studied in relation to figured worlds by analysing stories of participants in that world using an interactional positioning approach. Importantly, researchers analysing these stories must be familiar with the cultural worlds in which they are set. As an example, participants in a study of first- and second-year medical students in Norway recognised the contexts of learning in the two years as two different worlds. Their struggles to identify with the medical world were evident in some of their stories, and specific features of the sociocultural context were elaborated into their emerging professional identities (Vågan, 2011).

Social identity complexity

We all identify ourselves as belonging to multiple social groups. For example, the groups I identify with include women, researchers, mothers and medical doctors. These groups can be referred to as 'in-groups' and those with which I do not identify as 'out-groups'. Social psychologists have investigated how identification with multiple social groups can influence a person's perception of people who do not belong to any of their in-groups (Roccas & Brewer, 2002). When the groups with which a person identifies advocate conflicting attitudes and values, they are said to be *non-convergent*. The way we deal with non-convergence between our in-groups influences our own identity construction and how we relate to others.

The theory of *social identity complexity* describes four processes through which an individual can construct a social identity (Roccas & Brewer, 2002). The first is known as *intersection* and is associated with the least complex social identities. Those whose social identities follow this pattern identify only with other people who belong to all their own social groups. Those with a pattern called *dominance* identify strongly with only one of their in-groups and consider the others to be relatively unimportant. *Compartmentalisation* is a third, highly context-specific way of constructing a social identity. When such people are at work, for example, their professional identity is the sole basis of their categorisation of others; when in situations away from work, their perception of themselves in relation to others could be based on their other identities, such as their religion or ethnicity.

The fourth pattern is associated with the most complex social identity and described as *merger*. Other people are identified as in-group members if they are identified with any of that person's social groups, resulting in a more inclusive social identity. For people with this level of social identity complexity, in-group and out-group distinctions are minimised and bias against others reduced.

Many factors influence the complexity of a person's social identity, including life experiences, personal attributes and situational factors. Individuals are more likely to have complex social identities if they have grown up in a society that is multicultural, but not stratified along ethnic lines. Such people are likely to be more comfortable with ambiguity and uncertainty, to be open to change and to value tolerance above personal power. They tend to be more accepting of those who do not belong to any of their own social groups (Roccas & Brewer, 2002).

However, maintaining a complex social identity requires cognitive resources, and complexity may be diminished when there are increased demands on a person's attention. This includes situations where they are required to perform multiple concurrent tasks, work under increased stress or face a threat to one of their social groups. Medical professionals frequently experience these situations at work. Temporary reductions in social identity complexity can reduce a person's tolerance for ambiguity and uncertainty and their acceptance of people who do not belong to their own social groups (Roccas & Brewer, 2002). In later chapters I will discuss the relevance of this research in relation to my own findings, along with some implications for medical education and practice.

Modes of identification with social groups

Social psychologists have also investigated the different ways people identify with social groups (Roccas, Sagiv, Schwartz, Halevy, & Eidelson, 2008). This theory was originally derived from studies of patriotism and nationalism but has been applied to other groups whose members share common goals and a clearly defined membership. Understanding modes of group identification offers insight into how members of the medical profession respond when another doctor is criticised, or when they believe a colleague's actions to be inconsistent with the profession's values or expected standards.

A person's identification with a social group can be assessed in relation to four dimensions or modes: *importance* (how much I view the group as part of who I am); *commitment* (how much I want to benefit the group); *superiority* (how much I view my group as better than others) and *deference* (how much I honour, revere and submit to the group's norms, symbols and leaders). A profile can be built up for an individual, indicating how strongly each of these four modes of relating influences the degree to which they identify with a given group.

Importance and commitment together indicate a person's *attachment* to a group, while superiority and deference indicate their *glorification* of that group. Groups may require certain forms of identification, so that some groups may expect members to identify through glorification, while others may accept identification that is stronger on attachment (Roccas et al., 2008). *Critical attachment* is a form of group identification that is high on attachment and low on glorification (Roccas, Klar, & Liviatan, 2006). This mode of identification enables a group member to criticise or oppose an action of one of their in-groups if they believe it would violate the group's standards or values. For example, a person might oppose their nation entering a war even though its leaders support it, if he or she believes it would violate the nation's values.

This theory offers one explanation for the ways people react when members of a group with which they identify act in a way that conflicts with the group's values. A person who identifies more strongly through glorification is less likely to feel moral outrage towards members of their own group and more likely to defend their actions. Such people can morally disengage from the group's actions and support arguments that defend violations of expected moral standards. In contrast, those whose identification profile with respect to that group is stronger on attachment may find it easier to be critical. They are also more likely to experience a sense of guilt for their group's moral violations, and less likely to feel moral outrage towards members of other groups (Roccas et al., 2006). This is relevant to medical education because it enables us to consider the implications for the profession of different modes of identification.

Identity research in medical education

Socialisation, professionalism and identity construction

Learning to become a doctor presents social and emotional challenges as well as intellectual ones. As they observe and participate in clinical interactions, students discover that some patients arouse in them strong emotional responses, such as fear, disgust or desire, which they need to conceal or suppress. They are taught that clinicians must maintain an emotional distance from their patients. However, sometimes this can result in a failure of students to develop an awareness of their own emotional responses and to appreciate their potential influence on their own actions and those of others.

If this happens, it can impair their capacity to understand and acknowledge what a patient is experiencing, limiting the effectiveness of their therapeutic relationships. If this way of functioning spreads to their personal lives, it can be detrimental to their other relationships. Educators are faced with a challenge: to help students develop the capacity for a level of emotional awareness that is healthy and productive for a given situation (Bleakley et al., 2011). To meet this challenge, clinical teachers need to become aware of their own emotional responses and how to harness them productively in this context.

The focus of social research in medical education has shifted in recent years from socialisation to professional identity formation. This change signifies a new way of thinking about the social dimensions of medical education: one that highlights students' active involvement (DelVecchio Good, 2011; Holmes et al., 2011). Rather than focusing only on how people become doctors, researchers have also begun to inquire into what kinds of people emerge from contemporary clinical training and how students play an active part in their own identity construction.

In contemporary medical schools, there is often a strong emphasis on the concept of professionalism but a relative lack of attention to identity as a distinct, yet related phenomenon (Wilson, Cowin, Johnson, & Young, 2013). Professionalism involves displaying the behaviour of a professional, especially in areas such as ethics, expertise and service. Professional identity, on the other hand, is a form of occupational identity, relating to how people identify themselves and perform in that occupational role. It involves linking professional roles and competencies with values and aspirations and can be supported through ongoing self-reflection.

Contemporary work practices in health care often involve multidisciplinary teamwork. As a result, knowledge and power are distributed amongst team members rather than being held by one person. The potential benefits include increased transparency in decision-making as well as opportunities for more active patient participation. Within clinical teams, ongoing identity construction and reconstruction takes place as members are required to interact with each other about their work (Bleakley et al., 2011). However, for some experienced clinicians, this change raises disquiet about the erosion of their autonomy, and they may experience a sense of instability around their long-held professional identities.

The shift in emphasis in contemporary medical schools towards student-centred learning does not necessarily produce collaborative relationships between students and patients. When students begin to identify more with doctors than with patients as they advance in their training, there is a risk of increasing the social distance between students and patients and the potential for erosion of patient-centred attitudes (Bleakley & Bligh, 2008). In some circumstances, students may come to perceive patients as adversaries, whose interests are at odds with their own (Holmes et al., 2011). In this book, I will offer evidence of these adversarial relationships and consider what is at stake for clinical encounters when they are tacitly adopted.

Drama at the bedside

Despite the widespread discourse of patient-centredness in medical education, the relationship of prime importance in clinical teaching continues to be that between doctor and student (Bleakley & Bligh, 2008). Research into bedside teaching encounters in both hospital and primary care settings has confirmed that patients are often cast as material on which students learn (Monrouxe, Rees, & Bradley, 2009; Rees et al., 2013; Rees & Monrouxe, 2008). Because of the tendency to see patients in this way, opportunities to learn both from and with patients are not effectively utilised. These concerns are addressed by some of the new approaches advocated to redesign clinical teaching, learning and assessment (Bleakley & Bligh, 2008; Hodges, 2003).

Interactions between doctors, patients and medical students during bedside teaching encounters have recently become a focus of interest for empirical research. Participants in these interactions perform multiple roles, even though they may not be aware of doing so (Monrouxe et al., 2009). Using discourse analysis and dramaturgical theory to study how language generates meaning, insights have been gained into the way participants identify themselves in relation to those they are interacting with (Rees & Monrouxe, 2008). This in turn influences the way they represent characters in their stories and treat them in real life.

While patients may be involved as active participants at the beginning of bedside encounters, once the 'serious business of teaching' begins (Monrouxe et al., 2009, p. 923) they are often cast as a prop or *non-person*. The way people speak to each other, including the genre of language they use and changes in vocal tone, pitch and volume, is related to the roles people assume (Monrouxe et al., 2009; Rees et al., 2013; Rees & Monrouxe, 2008). For example, the way doctors or students speak to each other or the patient can include or exclude some of them from active participation, express differences in status, or create social distance. When doctors want to exclude the patient, they often use jargon and speak quietly and rapidly; this has been called 'back-stage talk' – using a dramaturgical term employed by Goffman (Monrouxe et al., 2009, p. 921). This is one of the ways in which doctors and students can be said to oscillate 'between two worlds: caring for the patient vs. teaching and learning medicine' (Monrouxe et al., 2009, p. 920).

Narrative-based activities in medical education

Narrative-based activities have been employed by medical educators to facilitate self-reflection and enrich students' professional identity formation. One group of researchers (Clandinin & Cave, 2008) worked with junior hospital doctors over a ten-week period using a narrative technique called the *parallel chart* (Charon, 2006). Participants wrote first-person stories about their clinical experiences and discussed them with peers in a facilitated group setting. They reported a range of benefits including helping them adjust to a new cultural setting, affirming the benefits of their existing approach or heightening their awareness of the complex nature of their work. The reflective process involved in constructing and sharing stories about a clinical experience contributes to identity formation, at the same time highlighting its narrative qualities.

Another study looked at clinical encounters of medical students and their mentors working in a free clinic for homeless people (Davenport, 2000). It revealed how they adopted shifting subject positions, associated with different identities in relation to patients. They learnt to alternate between witnessing a patient's illness experience and casting an objective medical gaze upon them.

Katz and Shotter (1996) developed and studied a practice they called *social poetics*. They found that clinicians who were focused on gathering diagnostic information often overlooked poetic moments: instances in which patients used figurative language such as metaphor to express their concerns or emotions. Researchers attended junior doctors' initial consultations and, immediately afterwards, joined junior doctors at conversations with their supervisors. They drew attention to poetic moments which had been overlooked by the junior doctor. When they returned to the patient, the potential significance of these communications was explored in relation to the clinical presentation, often with very productive results.

Over time, doctors participating in this project observed an improvement in their capacity to notice and interpret their patients' figurative language, and the emotional dimensions of their communication. These findings support the proposition that in order to function effectively, physicians must develop the capacity to move back and forth between different identities and subject positions (Bleakley et al., 2011). This is one manifestation of the unstable nature of identities that emerge in the workplace.

Another research collaboration taking a narrative approach to identity explored the experiences of medical students in their first clinical year by analysing their reflective writing portfolios (Pitkala & Mantyranta, 2003). The first clinical year can be an intensely emotional time for students, with rapid evolution in their identities as future doctors. Most students were able to reflect productively on their own internal conflicts, limitations and personal development. Narrative exercises such as these can help students recognise and derive meaning from key experiences, which in turn can support their professional identity development.

Relational perspectives

Some students in a Finnish study perceived patients as contributing to their identity development and reflected on how they imagined patients perceived them (Pitkala & Mantyranta, 2003). Some students believed that patients were more familiar with hospital culture than they were. When patients showed trust and confidence in them, this enhanced their identification as a doctor. This research highlights the relational nature of identity and the influence of patients upon medical students' identity formation, which is rarely identified in the literature.

A study of medical students in their first year of communication skills training investigated how they perceived their identities, and identified important influences (Vågan, 2009). They adopted a variety of different *conversation identities* as they interviewed volunteer patients. Students often thought that patients had different ideas about the meaning and purpose of an interaction from their own. When a student saw themselves as acting as a *professional*, they thought patients assumed they had greater knowledge than they actually did. On the other hand, when patients responded to them as if they were *lay conversation partners*, they would tell elaborate stories about their life, which students found frustrating when they were trying to elicit medical symptoms. Another conversation identity adopted by students was that of *trusted communication partner*. Students believed that when patients realised they had more time to listen to them, they would sometimes reveal information they had not confided to their doctors.

Participants in that study drew attention to the apparently irrelevant chatter of many of their patients. They did not reflect on why such stories are produced in this context, or their relevance for identity work. Also, only students' ideas about patients' perceptions of them could be considered, because patients were not interviewed. Nevertheless, it is interesting to note how students positioned themselves in relation to patients. The author concludes that it would be helpful for students to be guided to reflect on different types of conversation identities, to help them identify and adopt those likely to be most helpful in a given context (Vågan, 2009).

Critical discourse analysis was applied to ethnographic data gathered on an in-patient paediatric ward to explore students' use of language to construct patient roles and their own associated professional identities (Schrewe, Bates, Pratt, Ruitenberg, & McKellin, 2017). Thinking about student identities in relation to those constructed for the patients with whom they interact introduces a relational lens. In that study, discourses used to talk about patients typically characterised them either as a *disease category*, an *educational commodity* or a *marginalised actor*.

Identity dissonance

As mentioned earlier, identity is multiple in the sense that people identify with a number of social groups, including those defined by their gender, age, ethnicity or occupation (Iedema & Caldas-Coulthard, 2008). Some people find it easier to accommodate their emerging identity as a medical professional than others (Monrouxe, 2010). For many students, there is a perceived conflict between the expected values or performance of their emerging professional identity and those of their long-established identities, termed *identity dissonance* (Monrouxe, 2010). The reference to dissonance resonates with similar concepts described in relation to the *hidden curriculum* (Hafferty & Castellani, 2009) and the *dispositions* described as developing in students during their time in medical school (Sinclair, 1997). The construction of a professional identity might require some medical students to adopt a world view, emotional orientation or values which they perceive to be at odds with those of their established identities. Individuals from certain groups, including women, people from ethnic minorities and from less privileged socio-economic groups, are more likely to experience this sense of internal conflict (Monrouxe, 2010).

As an example of this phenomenon, one student told a story about her first experience of witnessing the death of a patient (Monrouxe, 2009). She was troubled by her perception that the emotional detachment expected of her professional self was inconsistent with her personal orientation to be emotionally expressive. Such experiences can precipitate emotional distress and lead some students to experience a loss of self-worth and uncertainty about their capacity to function effectively as a doctor. Dysfunctional coping mechanisms may result, including academic disengagement, substance abuse or other mental health problems (Monrouxe, 2010). Medical students as a group experience higher levels of distress and poorer mental health compared with other students or with the general population (Dyrbye et al., 2005). In order to enhance their health and well-being they need to be supported through the challenging process of identity construction, including being guided to recognise and reflect on experiences of dissonance.

Clinical case presentation genre

Many researchers have highlighted the importance of the clinical case presentation to the development of students' academic and professional identities (Anspach, 1998; Donnelly, 1997; Holmes & Ponte, 2011; Lingard, Garwood, Schryer, & Spafford, 2003; Lingard, Schryer, Garwood, & Spafford, 2003; Schryer, Lingard, & Spafford, 2005). They have explored how language is used by students or clinicians when reframing a patient's story as a clinical case. This process tends to depersonalise patients and cast doubt on the credibility of their account while enhancing that of the doctor (Donnelly, 1997). It is common in a case presentation to hear that the patient claims or denies something, but that a doctor confirms, or a scan report demonstrates something else. These terms imply that doctors and investigation reports are factual and not subject to human error or bias – which in fact, they are.

Genres are standardised linguistic templates that we use in everyday interactions which serve important functions in a community. They convey to newcomers how information is expected to be structured, and implicitly express common objectives of community members (Lemke, 2008). One of the functions of the case presentation genre is the management of uncertainty (Bleakley et al., 2011; Lingard, Garwood, et al., 2003). The tension between the requirements of a student and those of a working doctor in relation to case presentations can be understood as a clash between school and workplace communication genres (Lingard, Schryer, et al., 2003).

Naturally, students want to give the best possible impression of themselves in front of their teachers and peers. However, this could lead them to believe that any uncertainty they may feel should be concealed during case presentations. If this strategy carries over into a workplace setting, it could have dangerous consequences. Junior doctors need to inform their supervisors if the demands of a situation exceed their knowledge or competence. Educators could minimise the tendency to cover up uncertainty by being explicit about the different requirements of learning and practice settings (Lingard, Schryer, et al., 2003). They could also demonstrate to students that being open about what they do not know is a stimulus to learning, by modelling this behaviour in their own presentations and responding constructively to students' expressions of uncertainty.

When a student translates a patient's story into a case presentation, this act simultaneously transforms that person into a case and contributes to the student's identification as a medical professional (Holmes & Ponte, 2011). Contemporary research supports the idea of identity as a relational phenomenon, influenced by both intrinsic and extrinsic factors (Monrouxe, 2010). Innovative research methods employed in the study of medical students' identity formation include the collection of data using digital audio diaries, in which students record their experiences and reflections for later analysis (Monrouxe, 2009).

This book addresses several gaps in the literature. By including perspectives from students, patients and clinical teachers I have been able to study what kinds of identities are produced in relation to others through storytelling. Important knowledge about the perspectives of patients who participate in clinical teaching and how they experience their involvement has also been generated. The use of a dialogic approach to the analysis of the narrative data promotes an appreciation of the importance of power dynamics in clinical teaching interactions, which is seldom acknowledged in the literature or addressed in clinical teaching practice.

In the next chapter, I will provide details of the supporting theory for the study. I will take you into the field, sharing stories about my experiences as a physician-ethnographer and describe in detail how the research was designed and carried out.

References

Anspach, R. R. (1998). Notes on the sociology of medical discourse: The language of the case presentation. *Journal of Health and Social Behaviour, 29*(4), 357–375.

Bleakley, A. (2005). Stories as data, data as stories: Making sense of narrative inquiry in clinical education. *Medical Education, 39*(5), 534–540.

Bleakley, A., & Bligh, J. (2008). Students learning from patients: Let's get real in medical education. *Advances in Health Sciences Education, 13*, 89–107.

Bleakley, A., Bligh, J., & Browne, J. (2011). *Medical education for the future: Identity, power and location.* Dordrecht: Springer.

Charon, R. (2006). Chapter 8: The Parallel Chart. In *Narrative medicine: Honoring the stories of illness* (pp. 155–174). New York: Oxford University Press.

Chretien, K., Goldman, E., Craven, K., & Faselis, C. (2010). A qualitative study of the meaning of physical examination teaching for patients. *Journal of General Internal Medicine, 25*(8), 786–791.

Clandinin, D. J., & Cave, M.-T. (2008). Creating pedagogical spaces for developing doctor professional identity. *Medical Education, 42*, 765–770. doi:10.1111/j.1365-2923.2008.03098.x

Cruess, R. L., Cruess, S. R., Boudreau, D. J., Snell, L., & Steinert, Y. (2014). Reframing medical education to support professional identity formation. *Academic Medicine, 89*, 1446–1451.

Davenport, B. A. (2000). Witnessing and the medical gaze: How medical students learn to see at a free clinic for the homeless. *Medical Anthropology Quarterly, 14*(3), 310–327.

De Fina, A., Schiffrin, D., & Bamberg, M. (Eds.). (2006). *Discourse and identity.* Cambridge: Cambridge University Press.

De Peuter, J. (1998). The dialogics of narrative identity. In M. M. Bell & M. Gardiner (Eds.), *Bakhtin and the human sciences: No last words* (pp. 235). London: Sage.

DelVecchio Good, M.-J. (2011). The inner life of medicine: A commentary on anthropologies of clinical training in the twenty-first century. *Culture, Medicine and Psychiatry, 35*, 321–327. doi:10.1007/s11013-011-9217-z

Donetto, S. (2012). Talking about power in medical education. *Medical Education, 46*(12), 1141–1143. doi:10.1111/medu.12077

Donnelly, W. J. (1997). The language of medical case histories. *Annals of Internal Medicine, 127*(11), 1045–1048.

Dornan, T., Pearson, E., Carson, P., Helmich, E., & Bundy, C. (2015). Emotions and identity in the figured world of becoming a doctor. *Medical Education, 49*, 174–185. doi:10.1111/medu12587

Dyrbye, L., Thomas, M., & Shanafelt, T. (2005). Medical student distress: Causes, consequences and proposed solutions. *Mayo Clinic Proceedings, 80*(12), 1613–1622.

Frank, A. W. (2010). *Letting stories breathe: A socio-narratology.* Chicago, IL & London: University of Chicago Press.

Gardiner, M., & Bell, M. M. (1998). Bakhtin and the human sciences: A brief introduction. In M. M. Bell & M. Gardiner (Eds.), *Bakhtin and the human sciences* (pp. 1–12). London: Sage.

Garro, L. C., & Mattingly, C. (2000). Narrative as construct and construction. In C. Mattingly & L. C. Garro (Eds.), *Narrative and the cultural construction of illness and healing* (pp. 1–49). Berkeley, CA: University of California Press.

Goldie, J. (2012). The formation of professional identity in medical students: Considerations for educators. *Medical Teacher, 34*, e641–e648.

Guberman, R. M. (Ed.). (1996). *Julia Kristeva interviews.* New York: Columbia University Press.

Gubrium, J. F., & Holstein, J. A. (2009). *Analyzing narrative reality.* Los Angeles, CA: Sage.

Hafferty, F. W., & Castellani, B. (2009). The hidden curriculum: A theory of medical education. In C. Brosnan & B. S. Turner (Eds.), *Handbook of the sociology of medical education* (pp. 15–35). London & New York: Routledge.

Hodges, B. (2003). OSCE! Variations on a theme by Harden. *Medical Education, 37*, 1134–1140.

Holmes, S., Jenks, A., & Stonington, S. (2011). Clinical subjectivation: Anthropologies of contemporary biomedical training. *Culture, Medicine and Psychiatry, 35*, 105–112. doi:10.1007/s11013-011-9207-1

Holmes, S., & Ponte, M. (2011). En-case-ing the patient: Disciplining uncertainty in medical student patient presentations. *Culture, Medicine and Psychiatry, 35*, 163–182. doi:10.1007/s11013-011-9213-3

Holquist, M. (2002). *Dialogism* (2nd ed.). London & New York: Routledge.

Iedema, R., & Caldas-Coulthard, C. R. (2008). Introduction. In R. Iedema & C. R. Caldas-Coulthard (Eds.), *Identity trouble* (pp. 1–14). Houndmills: Palgrave Macmillan.

Katz, A. M., & Shotter, J. (1996). Hearing the patient's 'voice': Toward a social poetics in diagnostic interviews. *Social Science and Medicine, 43*(6), 919–931.

Lave, J., & Wenger, E. (1991). *Situated learning: Legitimate peripheral participation.* Cambridge: Cambridge University Press.

Lemke, J. L. (2008). Identity, development and desire: Critical questions. In C. R. Caldas-Coulthard & R. Iedema (Eds.), *Identity trouble: Critical discourse and contested identities* (pp. 17–42). Basingstoke & New York: Palgrave Macmillan.

Lingard, L., Garwood, K., Schryer, C. F., & Spafford, M. M. (2003). A certain art of uncertainty: Case presentation and the development of professional identity. *Social Science and Medicine, 56*, 603–616.

Lingard, L., Schryer, C., Garwood, K., & Spafford, M. (2003). 'Talking the talk': School and workplace genre tension in clerkship case presentations. *Medical Education, 37*, 612–620.

Middlebrook, C. (1996). *Seeing the crab: A memoir of dying.* New York: Basic Books.

Monrouxe, L. (2009). Solicited audio diaries in longitudinal narrative research: A view from inside. *Qualitative Research, 9*, 81–103. doi:10.1177/1468794108098032

Monrouxe, L. (2010). Identity, identification and medical education: Why should we care? *Medical Education, 44*(1), 40–49. doi:10.1111/j.1365-2923.2009.03440.x

Monrouxe, L., & Rees, C. (2015). Theoretical perspectives on identity: Researching identities in medical education. In J. Cleland & S. Durning (Eds.), *Researching medical education* (pp. 129–140). Oxford: Wiley-Blackwell.

Monrouxe, L., Rees, C., & Bradley, P. (2009). The construction of patients' involvement in hospital bedside teaching encounters. *Qualitative Health Research, 19*(7), 918–930. doi:10.1177/1049732309338583

Nair, B. R., Coughlan, J. L., & Hensley, M. J. (1997). Student and patient perspectives on bedside teaching. *Medical Education, 31*, 341–346.

Nelson, H. L. (2001) *Damaged identities: Narrative repair.* Ithaca, NY & London: Cornell University Press.

Pitkala, K. H., & Mantyranta, T. (2003). Professional socialization revised: Medical students' own conceptions related to adoption of the future physician's role—a qualitative study. *Medical Teacher, 25*(2), 155–160.

Rees, C., Ajjawi, R., & Monrouxe, L. V. (2013). The construction of power in family medicine bedside teaching: A video observation study. *Medical Education, 47*(2), 154–165. doi:10.1111/medu.12055

Rees, C., & Monrouxe, L. V. (2008). 'Is it alright if I-um-we unbutton your pyjama top now?' Pronominal use in bedside teaching encounters. *Communication and Medicine, 5*(2), 171–182.

Reissman, C. K. (2008). *Narrative methods for the human sciences.* Los Angeles, CA: Sage.

Rice, T. (2008). 'Beautiful murmurs': Stethoscopic listening and acoustic objectification. *The Senses and Society, 3*, 293–306. doi:10.2752/174589308X331332

Rimmon-Kenan, S. (2002). The story of 'I': Illness and narrative identity. *Narrative, 10*(1), 9–27.

Roccas, S., & Brewer, M. B. (2002). Social identity complexity. *Personality and Social Psychology Review, 6*(2), 88–106. doi:10.1207/s15327957pspr0602_01

Roccas, S., Klar, Y., & Liviatan, I. (2006). The paradox of group-based guilt: Modes of national identification, conflict vehemence, and reactions to the in-group's moral violations. *Journal of Personality and Social Psychology, 91*(4), 698–711.

Roccas, S., Sagiv, L., Schwartz, S., Halevy, N., & Eidelson, R. (2008). Toward a unifying model of identification with groups: Integrating theoretical perspectives. *Personality and Social Psychology Review, 12*(3), 280–306. doi:10.1177/1088868308319225

Schrewe, B., Bates, J., Pratt, D., Ruitenberg, C. W., & McKellin, W. H. (2017). The Big D(eal): Professional identity through discursive constructions of 'patient'. *Medical Education, 51*(6), 656–668. doi:10.1111/medu.13299

Schryer, C. F., Lingard, L., & Spafford, M. M. (2005). Techne or artful science and the genre of case presentations in healthcare settings. *Communication Monographs, 72*(2), 234–260.

Sinclair, S. (1997). *Making doctors: An institutional apprenticeship*. Oxford & New York: Berg.

Sools, A. (2013). Narrative health research: Exploring big and small stories as analytical tools. *Health: An Interdisciplinary Journal for the Social Study of Health, Illness and Medicine, 17*(1), 93–110. doi:10.1177/1363459312447259

Strawson, G. (2004). Against narrativity. *Ratio, 7*(4), 428–452. doi:https://doi.org/10.1111/j.1467-9329.2004.00264.x

Vågan, A. (2009). Medical students' perceptions of identity in communication skills training: A qualitative study. *Medical Education, 43*(3), 254–259. doi:10.1111/j.1365-2923.2008.03278.x

Vågan, A. (2011). Towards a sociocultural perspective on identity formation in education. *Mind, Culture, and Activity, 18*(1), 43–57. doi:10.1080/10749031003605839

Wenger, E. (1998). *Communities of practice: Learning, meaning and identity*. Cambridge: Cambridge University Press.

Wilson, I., Cowin, L. S., Johnson, M., & Young, H. (2013). Professional identity in medical students: Pedagogical challenges to medical education. *Teaching and Learning in Medicine, 25*(4), 369–373. doi:10.1080/10401334.2013.827968

Wortham, S. (2000). Interactional positioning and narrative self-construction. *Narrative Inquiry, 10*(1), 157–184. doi:10.1075/ni.10.1.11wor

Wortham, S. (2001). *Narratives in action: A strategy for research and analysis*. New York: Teachers College Press.

Wortham, S. (2006). *Learning identity: The joint emergence of social identification and academic learning*. New York: Cambridge University Press.

Wortham, S. (2008). The objectification of identity across events. *Linguistics and Education, 19*(3), 294–311.

2 Dialogues from the field

> Ethnographic texts are always dialogical – the site at which the voices of the
> other, alongside the voices of the author, come alive and interact with one
> another.
>
> (Denzin, 1997)

In this eloquent description, Denzin highlights the lively interaction between the
voices of the author and those of others that characterises ethnographic texts. In
the case of this book, my own voice is placed in dialogue with those of the study
participants – the patients, medical students and clinical teachers. In this chapter,
I open a window onto the research process and explain how these voices found
their way into the conversation. I describe the theoretical framework and
methods I used and how they align with each other and my position on knowledge and its production. I reveal some of my experiences as a novice ethnographer and reflect on my identities as physician and researcher. I describe the
participants, their recruitment, the sources of their stories and the contexts in
which they were told. I explain my analytic approach, including the selection
and analysis of stories, their assembly and juxtaposition, and the writing of the
ethnographic text.

Theoretical framework

Dialogue and the dynamic subject

My viewpoint on what counts as knowledge and how it can be produced is
informed by *critical post-structuralist* theory. According to this perspective,
social reality can only be observed indirectly, for example through dialogue,
stories or texts. The social reality we observe is inherently unstable because it is
reconstructed in everyday interactions. The critical aspect of this perspective
involves the consideration of power struggles and social contexts and their relationship with identity construction and performance (De Fina, Schiffrin, &
Bamberg, 2006).

The theoretical foundations of this research are based on the work of twen-
tieth century Russian cultural theorist, philosopher and literary critic Mikhail

Bakhtin (Gardiner & Bell, 1998). One of Bakhtin's many original ideas was that human relations are best understood as a *dialogue*, and this has shaped my way of thinking about identity and the clinical encounter. Bakhtin proposed that human *being* or existence – analogous to identity – is not something given to us, but rather an ongoing dialogic event that always takes place in relation to others (Holquist, 2002).

Thinking about human relations as a dialogue involves recognising that we construct and know ourselves only in relation to others. From a dialogic perspective, the production of meaning involves a creative struggle between *centripetal* forces tending to create unity and order and *centrifugal* forces tending towards ambiguity and chaos (Tanggaard, 2009). Although both verbal and non-verbal aspects of interactions are important, one of the fundamental ways we identify ourselves in relation to others is through storytelling.

Post-structuralist theorist and psychoanalyst Julia Kristeva further developed some of Bakhtin's ideas to propose a dynamic and relational view of the human subject, centred on the recognition of differences between oneself and the other (Guberman, 1996). She described the human subject as being *en procès* – a French term which is ambiguous, meaning both *in process* and *on trial*. The idea of *le sujet en procès* (the subject-in-process-and-on-trial) highlights the ongoing struggle and negotiation involved in the construction of subjects or identities (Prud'homme & Légaré, 2006). Consistent with Bakhtin's theoretical position on the tension between forces of order and chaos, Kristeva argued that the creative struggle for identity requires ordering, symbolic language as well as figurative, poetic language such as simile and metaphor.

One of the distinctive features of dialogic narrative analysis (sometimes called dialogic-performance narrative analysis) is the identification of multiple voices which are arranged and juxtaposed with each other. This process can be imagined as a kind of dialogue, which allows additional layers of meaning to emerge (Denzin, 1997). My approach combines aspects of dialogic methods developed by several authors, each of whom has acknowledged Bakhtin's influence (Gubrium & Holstein, 2009; Reissman, 2008; Frank, 2010; Wortham, 2000).

This analytic approach embodies Bakhtin's idea of the *multi-vocal* (many-voiced) nature of texts (Reissman, 2008). Within any interaction, multiple interpretations of an event can be expressed by a single narrator as well as by different participants (Tanggaard, 2009). In this book, I show how stories can also serve political ends and how some people's voices and stories are legitimised at the expense of others in less powerful positions (Denzin, 1997; Bosk, 1992). To give voice to those whose experiences are often marginalised or silenced, I include voices that are seldom heard, especially those of patients.

Ethnographic fieldwork

Ethnographic research involves researchers' sustained exposure to a particular cultural setting and its people. The process of gathering data from observations and interviews while immersed in a community is called *fieldwork*. Ethnographic methods were originally developed by anthropologists to study people from cultures they considered foreign to their own. However, they are now widely used to study social aspects of health and illness, including those within researchers' own cultural or social groups. Ethnography is ideal for gathering stories during casual interactions and formal interviews, and for appreciating the perspectives of both insiders and outsiders to that culture (Gubrium & Holstein, 2009).

Fieldwork involves close observation of material and social dimensions of everyday life, including those that are usually taken for granted (Murchison, 2010). Researchers in the field gather data about people, places and events using all their senses. Not only do they listen to their participants' words, but they also notice how they are spoken, their facial expressions and the sounds, smells and other ambient qualities of the environment in which the interaction is taking place. This allows them to construct detailed or 'thick' descriptions of the cultural environment (Liamputtong & Ezzy, 2005). To do this effectively, researchers need to develop an appreciation of the influence of contextual factors such as time, space and significant material objects and relationships. Ethnographic research allows insights to emerge that may not be revealed through participants' reports alone (Liamputtong & Ezzy, 2005). It is ideal for researchers studying the complexities of hospital life and the everyday practices of those who interact there as they work, learn or receive treatment and care (Long, Hunter, & van der Geest, 2008).

Ethnographic data has traditionally been recorded with hand-written field notes, although many contemporary ethnographers use audio or video recording technologies (Iedema, Long, & Forsyth, 2006; Liu, Manias, & Gerdz, 2012; Rees, Ajjawi, & Monrouxe, 2013). Ethnographers observe the outer world of people and events taking place in specific contexts, and the inner world of their own thoughts, feelings and physical sensations. These inner and outer worlds are brought together in the ethnographic text through analytic and reflective writing, both of which contribute to the production of meaning.

During my fieldwork, I observed students interviewing and examining patients under the watchful eyes of their clinical teachers. Sometimes, I became aware of shifts in my own way of seeing a patient, which affirmed the findings of an earlier ethnographic study at a clinic for homeless people (Davenport, 2000). I experienced this when I was watching a student carry out a neurological examination, observed by a tutor. As clinical signs were demonstrated or symptoms elicited, I found myself formulating a diagnosis for the patient's problem. The next moment, I became aware that he was looking bewildered or uncomfortable, and shifted my focus to an empathic witnessing of his experience.

The fieldwork begins

Finding my place

This was my first ethnographic project, and since it was undertaken for my doctoral research training, I saw myself as a novice researcher. I carried out my fieldwork in a large general hospital in Melbourne, the Australian city where I live. Having received formal approval from the relevant human ethics committees, I was welcomed by the clinical school director, who facilitated my access to potential participants. I attended the hospital two to three days a week for ten months – the duration of the 2010 academic year. I wondered, before starting the fieldwork, whether it might be difficult to limit myself to a research role, because I had worked for so many years as a hospital doctor. Some ethnographic researchers have successfully combined the roles of clinician and researcher at the same time (Berg, 1992; Sinclair, 1997). Due to my novice status as a researcher, I chose to minimise the blurring of these boundaries by carrying out the research in a hospital where I had never previously worked or studied.

For most of my career I had worked in rehabilitation hospitals, but I had visited acute hospitals regularly. Although I was familiar with them, I always felt like an outsider. I did not know my way around this particular hospital and in the early weeks I sometimes got lost. This tension between belonging and not belonging is useful in ethnographic research, offering insight into multiple perspectives. It was one of the parallels I observed between my own situation and that of the medical students in their first clinical year. Something else we shared was our home base at the hospital. I did not have access to office space so the only place I could store belongings that I did not want to carry with me, such as a coat or packed lunch, was the students' locker room.

My introduction to this space helped me find my place in the field and stimulated me to reflect on my new position. Julie, a member of the administrative staff, led me along a corridor and down some stairs to the basement. We passed the mail room, linen processing centre and uniform office before arriving at the students' locker room. Its walls were lined with rows of grey metal lockers. Many of the locker doors were damaged, and some looked as if they had been pried open with a crowbar. I chose a relatively intact one, and Julie applied a sticker with my name on it, stating that I was authorised to use it for the year. I attached the padlock I had brought with me, just as the students would when they arrived the following week.

This episode reminded me that my access to certain parts of the hospital was contingent on the goodwill of the clinical school director. Like the back-stage areas of a theatre, members of the public are not authorised to enter these spaces. It also highlighted the change in my status. In the past, as a consultant physician at the rehabilitation hospital where I worked, I had been responsible for patient care, junior medical staff supervision, and the co-ordination of a multidisciplinary team. I had my own office and access to administrative and support staff. Now, my home at the hospital was much humbler, consistent with my lowly and relatively tenuous position.

During the time I spent at the hospital, I came to appreciate the advantages of sharing a locker room with the students involved with my project. It seemed to reduce the social distance between us related to my qualifications, age and experience. It turned out to be a good place for informal contact with students. As we arrived in the morning or came to fetch food or books from the lockers, I could ask them about their plans for the day. I was often able to use these casual meetings to negotiate my attendance at a tutorial or ward round.

Another parallel between my experiences as a novice researcher and those of the medical students was the importance of negotiation. Students had to arrange tutorial times with their tutors and negotiate with patients before they could examine or talk with them. This contrasted with the highly structured teaching they had received at the university campus. As a researcher, I had to negotiate booking an interview room, contacting student or tutor groups and conferring with participants about their availability for an interview. Before attending a clinical teaching session, I had to contact students and tutors to find out when and where they were planned and ask if they would agree to me coming along. On the day, I had to gain agreement from patients and any non-participating students as well. The term *negotiated interactive observation* has been proposed to characterise fieldwork practices like these for researchers in health care settings (Wind, 2008).

Presence and impact

During my fieldwork, I sometimes wondered what other people made of my presence on the wards, and about my impact on that environment. Was I merely an observer or did I influence unfolding events? An incident that took place as I interviewed a patient on the ward made me realise that my presence would have had many subtle, unnoticed consequences. I had started my interview with Robin late in the morning and brought a chair to his bedside, so I could sit comfortably while we talked. About 15 minutes into the interview, his lunch arrived, and we took a break so he could eat.

When I returned, Robin explained that his doctors had visited on their ward round and that his interaction with them had been very different to those on previous rounds. Until now, he had not had a chance to talk to anyone about his concern that the aspirin he had been taking, prescribed by another doctor to prevent vascular disease, had caused bleeding from his stomach, which was the reason for his admission to hospital.

I asked him what was different about this interaction.

> Well, I think a lot of times things are said so fast that you can't absorb what it is. Like today it's been quite good. I tried to slow his pace down ... and he sat down and said: 'I really need to sit down'.

> So, how did you do that? How did you slow his pace down?

> Just by his manner, I think. He wanted to sit down, and I think he'd been on the go all the time, and for once he, sort of, sat down and actually heard what I was saying, because I was saying, like, that the aspirin has got to be the thing. And he said 'Yes, it is'.

> Do you think sitting down makes a difference?

> Oh, I think so, yeah.

So he sat down, and you had a proper discussion?

Yeah.

So, do you feel a bit clearer now, about what's going on and what it's all about?

Yeah. Normally ... they sort of stand at the end [of the bed] and sort of talk between [themselves].

So, they don't involve you very much in the discussion?

No, no.

How does that feel?

Oh, I mean – they've got a job to do, I suppose. [Sounds resigned]

Yeah. But you actually would prefer to get a bit more information?

Well it's good when the – I mean it was magic, because you brought the chair in and you sat down. Do you know what I mean? [Sounds animated]

Great. He wouldn't have, otherwise?

It wouldn't have been there if you hadn't come in.

This encounter between Robin and his doctor was apparently altered by the chair I had placed beside the bed, facilitating a more meaningful exchange. Before breaking for lunch, we had been talking about communicating with doctors and students, and this may also have helped Robin to bring up his concerns. This experience convinced me that my presence would have resulted in numerous small changes to the social and physical environment, with the potential for consequent effects on work, learning or patient care. I came to appreciate that my presence was a feature of the social context.

Strange but familiar

Ethnography was developed in the discipline of anthropology as a way of studying the cultures of people considered foreign or exotic by researchers. It was considered that researchers' unfamiliarity with the people they studied was an advantage, because aspects of culture embedded in everyday practices would be more visible than they would be to those belonging to that group (Geertz, 1973). My familiarity with hospitals could potentially have deprived this research of the quality of strangeness. However, other ethnographic projects have been carried out in hospital environments familiar to the researchers (Berg, 1992; Sinclair, 1997; Wind, 2008; Zaman, 2008). Choosing a field site in which I had never worked was a way of generating a sense of strangeness and unfamiliarity, as well as a strategy to avoid any misunderstandings about my role.

My professional background as a physician had several potential implications. One was the likelihood that assumptions would be made about my values and attitudes, and how I would interpret what I heard and witnessed. I was perceived as trustworthy, and this helped me gain acceptance from various gatekeepers, as well as potential participants. When students or tutors spoke frankly to me during interviews or elsewhere, I felt there was an implicit assumption that I would not portray my profession in a negative light to outsiders. This raised concerns for me that participants holding such assumptions might experience a sense of betrayal, if they were later revealed to be unfounded. Although I did provide critical interpretations of certain events, I avoided gratuitous revelations. I tried to empathise with narrators and story characters and avoid blaming individuals for what could be perceived as undesirable actions, by acknowledging the structural and cultural constraints of the context. However, it is important to acknowledge that my position on certain events entails value judgements.

My attitude towards my own identity as a physician-ethnographer evolved over the course of the fieldwork. Initially when I introduced myself, I downplayed my clinical background, although I never concealed it. This was partly to avoid any misunderstanding about my role, but also because I felt insecure about my emerging identity as a researcher. I was also concerned that if I were afforded privileges not available to other researchers, it would reduce my legitimacy in this role. However, I came to understand that my clinical background was an integral part of my identity as a researcher. I realised that participants were likely to feel more comfortable with my presence at the bedside, knowing that I was a doctor. As a result, I began to give this aspect of my identity more prominence, while making it clear I was there for research.

My familiarity with the technical language and practices of hospital medicine meant that I did not need to interrupt proceedings to clarify what participants were discussing. On the other hand, when I asked a participant questions to explore their perceptions of an event or practice, I was sometimes met with a look of disbelief that I would not already know the answers. I believe that my professional status was likely to have led to limitations in the data that I was able to collect. For example, as I discuss later, I felt that it contributed to the lack of opportunities I was offered to observe students interacting with patients on their own.

Other dimensions of my own identity were likely to have influenced the research, apart from my profession. These include my experience as a medical student and a clinical teacher, which helped me to understand the experiences and perspectives of those groups of participants. As well, I have lived with a chronic illness for most of my life, involving ongoing interactions with various doctors. The experiential knowledge gained from all these aspects of my own subjectivity influenced every stage of the research process, including my interpretations and the construction of the ethnographic text on which this book is based. For this reason, if another researcher had undertaken this project, neither the data gathered nor the interpretation of it would be identical with my own. It is characteristic of interpretative qualitative research methods, such as those employed in this project, that the findings are not *reproducible*, even though they would be expected to be *consistent* with those of another project using a similar approach to study similar research questions (Denzin, 1997).

Ethical considerations

As with any research involving human participants, I had to adhere to strict ethical guidelines so that the project could receive approval from the relevant human research ethics committees. Potential participants were given plain language statements and consent forms and I explained these in person before they gave their consent. Many participants were not interested in reading the forms, even though I encouraged them to do so, preferring to listen to my explanation and trust that I would do the right thing with their information.

However, it was important to look beyond procedural requirements when thinking about the project's ethical dimensions. Qualitative research can have unforeseen consequences for participants, so 'politics, moral issues and ethics infuse the research process in a way that procedural ethics can never address' (Liamputtong & Ezzy, 2005, p. 32). For example, there are complex ethical issues involved in recruiting hospital patients because of their vulnerable and dependent position. My first priorities were to avoid harm and minimise people's sense of obligation to participate. I explained that I was there only for research and was not part of the treating team. However, while interviewing one patient, he asked me about a team meeting that he assumed I had attended, and I realised he might not have understood or retained this explanation.

Privacy and confidentiality are important aspects of research ethics, which I have addressed in several ways. For the most part interviews were held in a private tutorial room, except for the patients. They were mostly interviewed in their bed in a shared ward, apart from one who was interviewed in his home. This lack of privacy was problematic and may have reduced some patients' willingness to discuss sensitive matters.

Ethical issues were also considered during the writing of research reports and papers about the project, including this book. The name of the hospital and university have not been disclosed. I have replaced participants' names with pseudonyms to minimise the risk of anyone being identified in reports or presentations. Where it could potentially have led to identification, I have changed or omitted other information. I chose names that reflected each person's gender and the region of origin of their actual names, to indicate the diversity of the participants' backgrounds. Most of the time students, teachers and patients called each other by their given names, but when anyone was addressed more formally, I maintained this form of address for their pseudonym.

As I chose which stories to include and how to tell them, I considered whether there could be any ramifications for those involved if the narrator or story characters were identified. Despite changing names and other details, the possibility remained that a participant might read a publication and recognise their own story. I weighed carefully any potential for harm against the significance of a story and the wider benefits of the research (Denzin, 1997).

When I was talking with my participants, and especially during the in-depth interviews, I was aware that an unexpected situation could arise that would require a prompt response. I cultivated *ethical mindfulness* as a preparation for such eventualities. This involved paying close attention to participants, as well as to my own sensations, perceptions and emotional responses (Guillemin & Heggen, 2008). This state of mindfulness would sometimes alert me to ethically important moments in an interaction. My evaluation of how the interaction was affecting a participant was guided by their demeanour, and I would also check my interpretation by asking whether they were feeling all right and were willing to proceed.

One particular interview with a student illustrates the importance of this kind of mindfulness. While we were discussing her educational background and work experience, she mentioned that she had been absent for an extended period from her medical course for health reasons. I continued with the interview without asking for details, but she referred to her health problem on two more occasions while we were discussing interactions with patients. At that point, I said that I would like to hear more about it, but only if she felt comfortable to tell me.

She explained the nature of her medical condition and how her experience of prolonged hospitalisation had profoundly affected her interactions with patients, especially those whose situation resembled hers in some way. Although she chose to reveal this information, speaking about it appeared to be causing her distress, as she had increasing difficulty speaking fluently and exhibited physical signs of anxiety. I decided to change the subject to something of a less personal nature, and she seemed happy to follow my lead, becoming calmer.

As I was winding up the interview, I took care to convey my gratitude, not only for her time and participation, but also for her willingness to reveal a very private part of her life to me. I assured her that no information identifying her, or the nature of her medical condition, would be revealed in any publications arising from the research. I encouraged her to contact me or the clinical school director if she experienced any ongoing distress or concerns.

During this interview, I was acutely aware of the importance of avoiding harm and affirming my participant's dignity and courage (Denzin, 1997). Throughout the time of my fieldwork, I strove to develop genuine connections with each participant, while respecting the proper boundaries of the relationship. I consider 'personal expressiveness, emotionality and empathy' as qualities to be cherished and celebrated within the research process (Denzin, 1997, p. 276). Whenever the interests of a participant and the data-gathering imperatives of the project appeared to be in conflict, I gave priority to those of the participant, even when this resulted in a missed opportunity to collect valuable data.

Recruiting the storytellers

Medical students

I recruited 20 students in their third year of a five-year undergraduate medical degree. Fifteen were interviewed twice, in first and second semester, and I accompanied them to ward rounds and bedside tutorials. Five other students, members of the tutorial groups of the original 15 students, were recruited later. Their formal consent to participation allowed me to describe what went on in tutorials more fully but they were not interviewed. I recruited students by email, promotional flyers and a presentation about my project as well as word-of-mouth through those already recruited. The sample was mainly one of convenience, but this approach has limitations, including the potential to unintentionally exclude certain groups and therefore miss out on useful data.

When I realised none of the first ten students enrolled in my study were men of Anglo-Australian background, despite this group making up a significant proportion of the cohort, I invited students meeting these criteria to participate. My eventual participant group came from diverse cultural backgrounds, with their families originating in East Asia, South-East Asia, South Asia, the Middle East and North Africa, as well as some with Anglo-Australian heritage. The 15 students interviewed comprised eight men and seven women between 20 and 22 years of age, most of whom had entered the course directly after leaving secondary school.

Students were recruited as individuals but received their clinical teaching in groups. Often at a bedside tutorial, only some of the students who were present were participants in my study. I informed all of them that only the words and actions of participants would be reported and offered to leave if anyone felt uncomfortable about my presence. I asked participants to discuss this with their peers outside the tutorial, in case they found it difficult to object in my presence. No objections were expressed but it is possible that some students with concerns were reluctant to voice them.

This was the first year of these students' immersion in real-life clinical practice after spending two years on pre-clinical studies, learning biomedical sciences and clinical skills, mostly practising with peers or simulated patients. In third year, most of their clinical interactions took place at hospitals with close links to their university medical school, but they also attended occasional community placements, exposing them to other clinical environments and models of care. Each student belonged to a group of ten for the year, rotating through a series of medical and surgical units for two to four weeks at a time. On each rotation, students' learning activities included ward rounds, outpatient clinics, operating theatre sessions and tutorials focused on specialist content. They were also urged to see patients on their own or in pairs, and carry out simple procedures under supervision, such as taking blood for pathology tests or inserting intravenous lines.

Assigned to each student group were two clinical tutors, one medical and one surgical. Each tutor met with the group weekly for teaching and practice of clinical skills, including interviewing and physical examination. They also had problem-based learning tutorials based on written clinical cases with mainly student-directed learning with guidance from another tutor. Additional tutorials focused on emergency procedures, communication for intimate examinations, and challenging interactions.

Clinical teachers

I recruited and interviewed seven clinical teachers involved with my student cohort. This was also a convenience sample. The two tutors who responded to my introductory email were particularly interested in teaching and enthusiastic about participating. My most successful strategy was to recruit tutors after attending their teaching sessions with my student participants. Before attending for the first time I would always seek their agreement, and afterwards I would invite them to join the study and participate in an interview. There were few women amongst the group of tutors involved with this student cohort, and there was only one woman recruited out of the seven clinical teacher participants. Like the students, the cultural backgrounds of the clinical teachers in my study were diverse: two were Anglo-Australian, one each from East Asia and South-East Asia, two from continental Europe and one from the United Kingdom. Some were fully trained consultants, but most were completing specialist training. There were four from medical specialty areas and one surgical trainee, one anaesthetist and pain specialist and one emergency physician.

Patients

Ethnographers are ideally placed to represent in their research the voices of those with little power and influence (Bosk, 1992; Denzin, 1997). The inclusion of patients as participants in this project was crucial because their voices and perspectives are rarely heard in this context. To participate, patients needed to be medically stable, alert, comfortable, and able to communicate in English, because I did not have access to interpreters. As a result, they resembled those usually favoured for teaching. This bias was inevitable to some extent, since only participants meeting these criteria could meaningfully consent and participate in an in-depth interview. I was unable to gather data from those who were more unwell, unable to speak English or had major cognitive difficulties, and I acknowledge that such patients may have had different experiences.

Often, I would identify someone on a tutorial or ward round who appeared suitable and would approach them afterwards to invite them to participate in the project. I would always gain verbal consent prior to observing their interactions in teaching sessions, but if they agreed to be interviewed, they would also be guided through the formal written consent process. Of the ten patients I approached this way, eight agreed to participate. I invited two other patients on the recommendation of students who had seen them in ward rounds or tutorials. In the final sample there were seven men and three women, seven of whom were in medical units and three in surgical units. There was less diversity of cultural background within the patient group: one was from East Asia, one from Eastern Europe, three from the United Kingdom and five of Anglo-Australian origin.

Gathering the stories

Stories gathered from field observations and interviews formed the largest and most important body of material. Seven students' reflective writing pieces were also included with their consent, along with written educational materials in the form of student and tutor handbooks.

Field observations: making contact

On two or three days a week during my fieldwork, I travelled for an hour by train from my home on the other side of the city to the hospital. I contacted students by text message or email or approached them in the locker room to ask about any teaching events I might attend. Their weekly bedside tutorials were valuable opportunities for gathering stories. Each tutorial involved interactions between a tutor and student group with several patients. Students also attended ward rounds and clinics, accompanying doctors in their everyday work, where up to 20 patients might be seen. At working ward rounds, students usually hovered in the background and rarely interacted with patients. However, doctors sometimes offered a brief explanation about a patient's condition, asked the students a question or two or invited them to observe an abnormal sign or perform a limited examination.

I recorded my observations of these events during and immediately afterwards using hand-written field notes, because I thought people might find the use of a recording device intimidating. My notes included information about non-verbal communication and my own impressions of other aspects of the context. The importance of senses other than sight and sound in building up a rich description of a setting and events is well recognised in ethnographic research. With well-written field notes, perceptions can be registered which would not be captured by recording technologies alone, such as a tense interpersonal atmosphere, sounds, odours, facial expressions or temperature in a space (Murchison, 2010).

However, the use of hand-written notes alone has limitations. The precise details of an interaction cannot be reliably captured, and as a result some analytic techniques which can be used on audio-recorded data cannot be applied to material recorded in this way. Despite the challenges, I was able to record sufficient detail to allow detailed descriptions and interpretations. I believe that my capacity for close observation and retention of detail, developed over many years of clinical work, helped me in this research context (Murchison, 2010). Other researchers have successfully employed audio and video recording devices in hospital settings, resulting in valuable additional data (Iedema et al., 2006; Liu et al., 2012; Monrouxe, Rees, & Bradley, 2009).

Unfortunately, there were gaps in the observational data I was able to collect. Before starting the fieldwork, I expected to spend a lot of my time accompanying students when they went to see patients on their own or in pairs, without a tutor. They were encouraged to do this as much as possible, to practise their skills. Apart from one occasion when I accompanied three students seeing a patient, I was only able to learn about these interactions indirectly, through interviews or conversations.

There are several potential explanations for this situation. Firstly, I was only at the hospital for two or three days each week, and although I asked students to contact me when they were going to see a patient, these interactions were often spontaneous and might have taken place when I was not there. Secondly, I imagined that some of them were not doing much practice on their own, and they later confirmed this. However, I believe there was a third reason for my lack of access to these sessions. During our interviews, several students described differences between how they related to patients when a doctor was present and when they were on their own. Because I was both a researcher and a doctor, my presence at these sessions would have fundamentally changed them and students might have preferred to avoid this.

Handbooks: espoused values and expected practices

As previously discussed, there are tensions between the values espoused by the medical school and some of the practices and attitudes students observe in clinical settings. This is often discussed in terms of a tension between official teaching and the hidden curriculum (Hafferty & Castellani, 2009; Lempp & Seale, 2004; Browning, Meyer, Truog, & Solomon, 2007). I obtained copies of handbooks produced for students and tutors as a guide to the year's teaching and learning activities. These texts represented the espoused values and practices expected of students in their interactions with patients. They helped me to establish how some everyday practices were consistent with the values advocated by the clinical school, while others seemed incompatible with them.

Interviews: fertile ground for storytelling

I carried out 47 in-depth, semi-structured interviews, resulting in a large body of narrative material. I recorded the interviews on a small digital audio device, supplemented with written notes about the environment and non-verbal aspects of the interaction. Each student was interviewed in the first and second semesters and patients and clinical teachers were each interviewed once. Student and teacher interviews took place in a quiet tutorial room, while patients were interviewed at their bedside. I tried to offer some privacy by closing the curtains around the bed, but our conversations could have been heard by others and sounds from the ward environment were often audible. The interviews were conversational in style, but I also had an interview guide as a prompt.

After they had been transcribed verbatim, I reviewed each transcript while listening to the audio file to correct errors and add notes about non-verbal aspects of the interaction, such as laughter and the tone or volume of voices. I included hesitations, interruptions and my own contributions as well as those of participants, because stories are always co-constructed, in this case between researcher and participant (Reissman, 2008). This provided information as to what may have prompted the telling of particular stories, adding to the richness of the data and contributing to the analysis. I was given permission to include reflective essays written by some of the students; these contained interesting stories, but none of them were included in the final text.

Some authors have argued that interview data only represents what people say they do, as opposed to what they actually do. However, I see them as an integral part of the fieldwork: a site in which narratives are constructed dialogically (Vickers, Zychowicz, & Morones, 2010; Kvale, 2006; Reissman, 2008; Tanggaard, 2007, 2009; Wortham, 2000). The stories produced and performed in these interviews are not already in the mind of the participant; instead, they emerge from the unique interaction between researcher and participant in that context. Often during these interviews, speaking about an event seemed to make the participant aware of something for the first time.

During my interview with Yong, a clinical tutor and surgical trainee, I asked him to reflect on how doctors create distance from patients or make connections with them. This was one of my earliest research interviews and I put the question in a rather clumsy way, but even so Yong's response was interesting.

What strategies, what … helps to create a distance, when you feel you need to do that? How do you go about that?

Umm – [pause] I haven't really formalised a strategy! [Laughter]

I know – I mean, we're talking about things we don't normally articulate – we just do them, but I guess for my purposes, it's interesting to try and articulate that.

Yeah. One – I think the way, sort of, I tend to, you know – for patients when you – [pause] now I think about it, for patients that you want them to – for the patient you're sort of trying to make a connection, you tend to – or I tend to – listen more, and just wait for them to tell me things. But whereas when I'm trying to distance myself I just ask, 'this and this' – and just – I just ask questions, once I've got my answers, and then I say 'OK, that's fine', and we just move on to the next patient, so – trying to keep things simple, and just direct. [Tapping his pen on the table with the words 'distance', 'ask', 'this' and 'this'] Whereas when you, sort of, wanting to – know a bit more about the patient, to establish some sort of connection then – [pause] – then you just – more likely to stand there or sit there and give a bit of time. Even different – sometimes you can sit down with the patient. But other times if you really – I think it's reflected in your body language – you tend to start to move away, look aside, and pick up another person's [file] – the next patient …'

Yes, you're just showing, you know, 'I don't want to be here anyway' [laughter], you're moving on …

So – you're moving on. And then that's sort of how – how it sort of happens, in the ward.

In response to my question about creating distance or connection, Yong's speech became slow and hesitant, with many long pauses, whereas otherwise he was very fluent, having been educated in Australia. His response illustrates how interviews can provide opportunities for reflection on everyday practices. His use of the phrase: 'now I think about it' and his closing remark: 'that's sort of how – how it sort of happens, in the ward' suggest that during the interview, he became aware of things he had been doing in an unreflective way.

Dialogic narrative analysis

Taking a dialogic approach to the narrative analysis involved considering not only a story's content, but also the way it had been constructed and told within a given context, and to consider the contributions of all those involved. I had to identify and maintain differences between individual stories, rather than mini-mising them in the pursuit of common themes. This approach also involved drawing links and connections within stories, as well as juxtaposing different stories, which can generate knowledge that is unavailable through the use of other analytic methods.

The version of dialogic narrative analysis used for this project was developed by adapting the approach of Gubrium and Holstein (2009), incorporating insights from Reissman (2008) and Frank (2010). I also employed a technique known as *interactional positioning* (Wortham, 2000) to enrich and extend my interpretations. I describe the process here in detail so it will be easier to grasp its application to the stories in later chapters.

Preliminary steps

A large volume of material was gathered during my fieldwork, and since nar-rative analysis is an intensive and time-consuming process, it was not feasible to apply it to all the data. I needed to select stories for analysis, from which I would choose those for inclusion in the ethnographic text. My definition of a story for this purpose included passages of interactive talk without any formal narrative structure. As mentioned in the previous chapter, I often use the terms *narrative* and *story* interchangeably, except that I use narrative when referring to more theoretical considerations about stories and storytelling and I refer to a particular account as a story. In a story, there is a consequential relationship between events that are described; in other words, something happens as a result of an earlier event. A story also tells the audience something about the character of people whose actions are described. There is often some kind of trouble or dis-turbance to the expected course of events, resulting in suspense and ultimately, resolution and evaluation of events and story characters (Frank, 2010).

Before selecting stories for analysis, I reviewed the entire body of data mul-tiple times. This process of review overlapped in time with the data collection and involved many hours of listening to audio recordings and closely reading field notes and transcripts. During this process I began to notice connections between certain stories, for example those that focused on certain types of experiences, and subsequently assembled them into tables and charts. These stories became candidates for analysis, and those which made significant and original contributions to the findings were included in the final text.

Some stories were selected because they related to a unique situation or revealed a new perspective on the research question. Others provoked a strong emotional response in me, such as surprise, disappointment or anger. My reflections on these responses can be understood as a way of thinking with stories, whereas the analytic process is a way of thinking about stories (Bleakley, 2005; Frank, 2004). Working with the data, I appreciated how stories exercise a form of agency: by provoking responses in those who receive them, thereby influencing events in the social world (Frank, 2006).

The analytic process involved paying attention to several dimensions of a story: contexts, production, performance and work. I worked through each story several times considering each aspect in turn. Subsequently, the findings from these steps were integrated by assembling and juxtaposing related stories, revealing additional layers of meaning.

Narrative contexts

When analysing stories told during a research interview about clinical encounters, there are multiple sets of contexts to be considered. We can think of them as being contained within each other, like a set of Russian nesting dolls. In the centre are the *narrated events*: the encounters being described by the storyteller, which are contained within the interview or clinical encounter, which can be described as a *storytelling event* (Reissman, 2008). In turn, the interview or encounter is contained within a further storytelling event, such as this book, and each layer has its own set of contexts. Narrative contexts include the time, place and physical environment, and social contexts including relationships between people involved.

Another dimension of narrative context is *intertextuality*, a term coined by Kristeva (Guberman, 1996). It relates to the idea that words, ideas and plots from narratives embedded in particular cultural groups are woven, deliberately or unconsciously, into new stories told by people belonging to those groups (Gubrium & Holstein, 2009). A tale can be constructed from other stories or refer explicitly to them, especially when talking about shared experiences in a particular context (Gubrium & Holstein, 2009). Familiar narratives shape the way audiences or readers interpret a story being told in the present moment. Along with the idea of intertextuality, the term *resonance* has been used to express the idea that 'stories echo other stories ... and are also told to be echoed in future stories' (Frank, 2010, p. 37).

Narrative production

I began by considering *narrative elicitation* or, in other words, what prompted the telling of a story, for example, a question or an idea expressed earlier.

I noted the degree to which the people interacting collaborated: whether they shared power and control over the emerging story or whether one speaker dominated. When observing an interaction at a bedside tutorial, I noted when someone said or did something that interfered with another person's storytelling. When an emerging story is 'disrupted, pre-empted, ignored [or] shut down', this can be described as *narrative suppression* and is a manifestation of the power dynamics of the interaction (Gubrium & Holstein, 2009, p. 52).

I looked for evidence of *linkages* or associations between one idea and another that were uncovered by the way the story was told. A patient's story sometimes revealed their personal associations between their present illness and prior life events (Gubrium & Holstein, 2009). The metaphorical expressions employed by a narrator could reveal how they thought about abstract concepts (Kövecses, 2010).

The way a narrator used pronouns or verb tenses can point to certain subtle meanings in a given context (Wortham, 2001). For example, the use of first-person singular pronouns 'I' and 'me' tends to highlight individual responsibility. In contrast, the use of first-person plural pronouns 'we' and 'us' to refer to a narrator's own actions implies that responsibility is shared with others. As in the analysis of Daniel's story in the first chapter, I also paid attention to the way speakers positioned themselves interactionally in relation to other people or social groups (Wortham, 2000). This also drew attention to the power dynamics of an interaction.

Narrative performance

Since every story is designed and staged for a particular audience, I paid attention to the performative aspects of storytelling, in interviews and clinical teaching encounters. This included the relative positions in space of those interacting, their modes of dress, use of props or objects, facial expressions and gestures. Vocal volume, intonation and emphasis were also aspects of performance which contributed to the production of meaning (Gubrium & Holstein, 2009; Reissman, 2008).

Within any language, there are different forms of expression – described as *voices* – that are characteristic of particular social groups (Wortham, 2001). When a speaker is represented as using a certain voice, it means that their words indicate a particular social position or membership of a cultural group (Wortham, 2001). Bakhtin called this property of language *heteroglossia*, contending that: 'All words have the 'taste' of a profession, a genre, a tendency, a particular work, a particular person, a generation, an age group, the day and hour' (Bakhtin, 1981, p. 293).

Within any storytelling event, a narrator will often use multiple voices when speaking for themselves and others to position themselves with respect to story characters and audiences. This narrative device is characteristic of novelistic writing but is also common in everyday interactions. The concept of *double voicing* refers to the idea that speakers convey something about people and events 'not only by representing objects but also by positioning themselves with respect to others who have spoken about the same objects' (Wortham, 2001, p. 63). A narrator speaks through the voice of another person when he or she represents or refers to another's speech in a particular way. They are said to be double voicing because they convey their own point of view indirectly by representing the speech of others in certain ways.

A related concept is that of *ventriloquation*, which refers to 'the process of positioning oneself by juxtaposing and speaking through others' voices' (Wortham, 2001, p. 67). When a narrator represents a story character as having spoken certain words, even if it is made to sound like a direct quote, they are in fact controlling what the character says, and how it is said, just as a ventriloquist controls their mannequin. Through ventriloquation, narrators position themselves closer to, or distance themselves from, their story characters (Wortham, 2001).

Narrative work

The next step required me to consider the story as a whole and the work accomplished by the act of telling it. This included how it was received and the consequences of telling it in that context (Frank, 2010; Reissman, 2008). Because of my interest in identities and the relational aspects of storytelling encounters, I was especially interested in how narrators positioned themselves in the story to convey something about their own character (Reissman, 2008; Monrouxe, 2010).

I revisited the question of power relations at this stage, and how they were enacted through storytelling. This was often related to social relationships between narrators, audiences and story characters, as discussed when considering narrative contexts. Fears and desires can often be inferred as motivating forces for people's actions, even when they are not acknowledged. Identifying fears and desires provided potential explanations for some actions of story characters and narrators' evaluations of them (Frank, 2004, 2010). I also took note of inconsistencies and contradictions as well as absences – occasions where something remained unsaid that I might have expected to be mentioned (Gubrium & Holstein, 2009). I considered whether the responses of audiences or collaborators indicated that they respected the authority of a storyteller, and whether the story appeared to have served its intended purpose (Gubrium & Holstein, 2009).

Stories in dialogue

To compose Chapters 3 to 7 of this book, I assembled stories that addressed a particular theme or dimension of the data from different perspectives. I placed the stories and their narrators *in dialogue* with each other by juxtaposing them and considering them in relation to each other. This enabled a further level of analysis, not only representing diverse perspectives but also highlighting differences between them. An ongoing, iterative process of analysis and interpretation continued during the writing of the ethnographic text.

In the next chapter, I consider the differences observed by students between real patients and the simulated encounters that they have previously participated

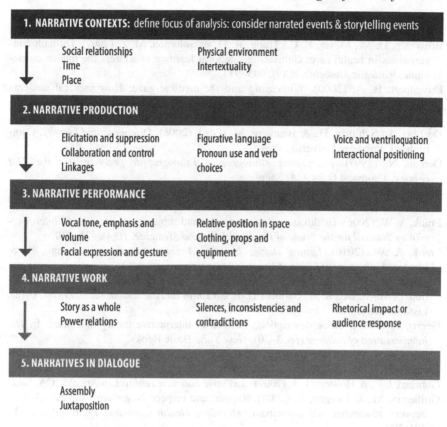

1. NARRATIVE CONTEXTS: define focus of analysis: consider narrated events & storytelling events

Social relationships
Time
Place

Physical environment
Intertextuality

2. NARRATIVE PRODUCTION

Elicitation and suppression
Collaboration and control
Linkages

Figurative language
Pronoun use and verb
choices

Voice and ventriloquation
Interactional positioning

3. NARRATIVE PERFORMANCE

Vocal tone, emphasis and
volume
Facial expression and gesture

Relative position in space
Clothing, props and
equipment

4. NARRATIVE WORK

Story as a whole
Power relations

Silences, inconsistencies and
contradictions

Rhetorical impact or
audience response

5. NARRATIVES IN DIALOGUE

Assembly
Juxtaposition

Figure 2.1 Dialogic narrative analysis.

in during their communication skills training, prior to entering the clinical setting. One student uses multiple voices to tell a story about her struggle for an integrated identity. My analysis of a bedside teaching encounter demonstrates how a patient's story, elicited during a history-taking interview, can accomplish substantial identity work. This provides a clue to the meanings that can emerge from stories told by patients, even when students and their teachers consider them to be irrelevant or tangential to the purpose of the interaction.

References

Bakhtin, M. M. (1981). Discourse in the novel (C. Emerson & M. Holquist, Trans.). In M. Holquist (Ed.), *The dialogic imagination* (pp. 59–422). Austin, TX: University of Texas Press.

Berg, M. (1992). The construction of medical disposals: Medical sociology and medical problem solving in clinical practice. *Sociology of Health and Illness, 14*(2), 151–180.

Bleakley, A. (2005). Stories as data, data as stories: Making sense of narrative inquiry in clinical education. *Medical Education, 39*(5), 534–540.

Bosk, C. (1992). *All God's mistakes: Genetic counselling in a pediatric hospital.* Chicago, IL: The University of Chicago Press.

Browning, D. M., Meyer, E. C., Truog, R. D., & Solomon, M. Z. (2007). Difficult conversations in health care: Cultivating relational learning to address the hidden curriculum. *Academic Medicine, 82*(9), 905–913.

Davenport, B. A. (2000). Witnessing and the medical gaze: How medical students learn to see at a free clinic for the homeless. *Medical Anthropology Quarterly, 14*(3), 310–327.

De Fina, A., Schiffrin, D., & Bamberg, M. (Eds.). (2006). *Discourse and identity.* Cambridge: Cambridge University Press.

Denzin, N. (1997). *Interpretive ethnography: Ethnographic practices for the 21st century.* Thousand Oaks, CA: Sage.

Frank, A. W. (2004). Asking the right question about pain: Narrative and phronesis. *Literature and Medicine, 23*(2), 209–225.

Frank, A. W. (2006). Health stories as connectors and subjectifiers. *Health: An Interdisciplinary Journal for the Study of Health, Illness and Medicine, 10*(4), 421–440.

Frank, A. W. (2010). *Letting stories breathe: A socio-narratology.* Chicago, IL & London: University of Chicago Press.

Gardiner, M., & Bell, M. M. (1998). Bakhtin and the human sciences: A brief introduction. In M. M. Bell & M. Gardiner (Eds.), *Bakhtin and the human sciences* (pp. 1–12). London: Sage.

Geertz, C. (1973). Thick description: Toward an interpretive theory of culture. In *The interpretation of cultures* (pp. 3–30). New York: Basic Books.

Guberman, R. M. (Ed.) (1996). *Julia Kristeva interviews.* New York: Columbia University Press.

Gubrium, J. F., & Holstein, J. A. (2009). *Analyzing narrative reality.* Los Angeles, CA: Sage.

Guillemin, M., & Heggen, K. (2008). Rapport and respect: Negotiating ethical relations between researcher and participant. *Medicine, Health Care and Philosophy, 12*(3), 291–299.

Hafferty, F. W., & Castellani, B. (2009). The hidden curriculum: A theory of medical education. In C. Brosnan & B. S. Turner (Eds.), *Handbook of the sociology of medical education* (pp. 15–35). London & New York: Routledge.

Holquist, M. (2002). *Dialogism* (2nd ed.). London & New York: Routledge.

Iedema, R., Long, D., & Forsyth, R. (2006). Visibilising clinical work: Video ethnography in the contemporary hospital. *Health Sociology Review, 15*(2), 156–168.

Kövecses, Z. (2010). *Metaphor: A practical introduction* (2nd ed.). New York: Oxford University Press.

Kvale, S. (2006). Dominance through interviews and dialogues. *Qualitative Inquiry, 12*(3), 480–500. doi:10.1177/1077800406286235

Lempp, H., & Seale, C. (2004). The hidden curriculum in undergraduate medical education: Qualitative study of medical students' perceptions of teaching. *British Medical Journal, 329*, 770–773.

Liamputtong, P., & Ezzy, D. (2005). *Qualitative research methods* (2nd ed.). Melbourne: Oxford University Press.

Liu, W., Manias, E., & Gerdz, M. (2012). Medication communication during ward rounds on medical wards: Power relations and spatial practices. *Health (London), 17*(2), 113–134. doi:10.1177/1363459312447257

Long, D., Hunter, C., & van der Geest, S. (2008). When the field is a ward or clinic: Hospital ethnography. *Anthropology and Medicine, 15*(2), 71–78.

Monrouxe, L. (2010). Identity, identification and medical education: Why should we care? *Medical Education, 44*(1), 40–49. doi:10.1111/j.1365-2923.2009.03440.x

Monrouxe, L., Rees, C., & Bradley, P. (2009). The construction of patients' involvement in hospital bedside teaching encounters. *Qualitative Health Research, 19*(7), 918–930. doi:10.1177/1049732309338583

Murchison, J. M. (2010). *Ethnography essentials*. San Francisco, CA: Jossey-Bass.

Prud'homme, J., & Légaré, L. (2006). The subject in process. *Signo*. Retrieved from www.signosemio.com

Rees, C., Ajjawi, R., & Monrouxe, L. V. (2013). The construction of power in family medicine bedside teaching: A video observation study. *Medical Education, 47*(2), 154–165. doi:10.1111/medu.12055

Reissman, C. K. (2008). *Narrative methods for the human sciences*. Los Angeles, CA: Sage.

Sinclair, S. (1997). *Making doctors: An institutional apprenticeship*. Oxford & New York: Berg.

Tanggaard, L. (2007). The research interview as discourses crossing swords: The researcher and apprentice on crossing roads. *Qualitative Inquiry, 13*(1), 160–176.

Tanggaard, L. (2009). The research interview as a dialogical context for the production of social life and personal narratives. *Qualitative Inquiry, 15*(9), 1498–1515.

Vickers, C. H., Zychowicz, S., & Morones, J. R. (2010). Living with pain: Narrating an ideological position toward healthcare. *Communication and Medicine, 7*(1), 85–92.

Wind, G. (2008). Negotiated interactive observation: Doing fieldwork in hospital settings. *Anthropology and Medicine, 15*(2), 79–89.

Wortham, S. (2000). Interactional positioning and narrative self-construction. *Narrative Inquiry, 10*(1), 157–184. doi:10.1075/ni.10.1.11wor

Wortham, S. (2001). *Narratives in action: A strategy for research and analysis*. New York: Teachers College Press.

Zaman, S. (2008). Native among the natives: Physician anthropologist doing hospital ethnography at home. *Journal of Contemporary Ethnography, 37*, 135–154.

3   Real patients are different

It's a very different world taking a history from a patient, compared to doing it with your fellow students. Real patients don't know what you actually want to hear; you have to specifically get it out of them. … They'll start on one thing and they'll end up talking about their grandson and you're like: 'OK – I'm really going to have to cut you off!' But I've got to admit that I often just let them keep going because, you know, like – I've got stacks of time, and I don't take eight histories a day, and I'm not pressed for time … and once they've finished, I just steer the conversation back.

Andrew, medical student

Learning about clinical communication

The focus of this chapter is on students' perception that many patients tell stories during medical interviews that cause them to deviate from their expected course. I present and analyse one student's story about how a clinical tutor advised her to respond in such situations, which reveals the creative struggle to integrate her emerging and more established identities. Through the analysis of an excerpt from a bedside tutorial, I demonstrate how story fragments about a patient's life are interwoven with the history of his illness. These self-identifying stories serve important functions, although they are often overlooked or deliberately excluded from the presentation of the case.

Learning how to communicate effectively with patients occupies a significant part of the curriculum in medical schools these days. In the early stages of their training, students are taught to develop a systematic approach to diagnosing a patient's condition. They learn which questions to ask in relation to each body system, and how to examine the relevant parts of the body. Symptoms, such as pain or a change in bodily function, may be volunteered by patients or discovered as the student asks questions in the clinical interview, signified by the expression *taking the history*. Signs observed during the physical examination might include swelling of a joint, weakness of a muscle or an abnormal heart sound. Students also learn about clinical reasoning: the process by which doctors integrate the information from their history and examination findings, often supplemented by investigation results. Through clinical reasoning, they develop a list of possible explanations for the patient's presentation, known as the differential diagnosis. They know that they will be expected to reconstruct the story in a way that points towards the most likely diagnosis. This is an important skill they need to develop and is part of learning to think like a doctor.

Some approaches to the teaching of clinical communication skills can lead students to focus excessively on the instrumental aspects of the interaction. Sometimes they are provided with lists of things they should and should not do or say. For example, a student may be told to show attentiveness by leaning towards a patient and maintaining eye contact. However, this can come across as insincere or stilted if they do not genuinely pay attention to what the patient is saying or respond to contextual cues, including patients' verbal or non-verbal expressions of emotion. Communication is an inherently creative endeavour and its meaning is defined by subjective experience rather than instrumental skills (Salmon & Young, 2011).

Medical students have some contact with patients in the early stages of their course, but this may be very limited. Often, they practice history-taking and physical examinations on fellow students. Sometimes they have access to *simulated patients*: people trained to perform the role of a person presenting with a particular condition. This is considered a safe and supportive environment for learning, acting as a bridge between the classroom and authentic health care settings (Bligh & Bleakley, 2006). However, there are potential problems with relying too heavily on substitutes for real patients as students begin to learn these skills (Bligh & Bleakley, 2006; Hanna & Fins, 2006). Andrew's story at the start of this chapter illustrates how it can lead students to expect patients to give the story of their illness in an orderly fashion, when in reality it often emerges in quite a messy way.

Andrew's reflection on patients' tendency to ramble during history-taking interviews shows that he finds it both amusing and exasperating. It presents a challenge because he has to work hard to uncover the information he needs to make a diagnosis. He is willing to listen to their stories, but implies that when he becomes a doctor, he will not have time. For many students, it is difficult to overcome a long-held belief that it is rude to interrupt people. They can feel torn between wanting to be polite and needing to gather certain information, and struggle to redirect a patient without appearing abrupt.

These observations led me to reflect on several questions. Why do patients tell stories that seem irrelevant or tangential? Is it just because they don't know what is relevant, or could there be something else going on? What can we find out by listening to their stories, and what is lost when we don't? To explore these questions, I needed to think about what was accomplished when a particular story was told in a given context. I asked students to talk about their interactions with patients and compare them with the simulated and peer interactions they were familiar with prior to starting at the hospital. I noticed that many of them employed metaphorical expressions when they did so.

Storytelling metaphors

Metaphors are ubiquitous, populating our everyday conversations and shaping the way we perceive the world and act within it (Kövecses, 2010; Lakoff & Johnson, 1980). Metaphorical concepts are often rooted in embodied experience; for example, the expression *boiling with rage* reflects the bodily sensation of heat and the agitation associated with extreme anger. The use of a metaphorical expression offers a way of understanding an abstract concept by representing it in terms of a more concrete one (Kövecses, 2010). Metaphors offer clues as to how the speaker conceptualises the domain of experience in question; they may be used either habitually or rhetorically (Kövecses, 2010; Rees, Knight, & Wilkinson, 2007). The choice of metaphor highlights some aspects of a concept while obscuring others. In this way, it can influence the way people understand the corresponding abstract concept (Kövecses, 2010; Lakoff & Johnson, 1980). Identifying the metaphorical expressions employed by students to talk about their interactions with patients can improve our understanding of the meanings they ascribe to them (Rees et al., 2007).

To explore this idea further, I analysed the student interview data to determine which metaphors students employed when talking about their interactions with patients. The common expressions revealed the conceptual understandings behind those metaphors (Kövecses, 2010; Rees et al., 2007). A small number of students spoke of their interviews with real patients as needing to be more fluid or flexible than those they had experienced with peers or simulated patients, which were characterised as being more rigid. These expressions represent the interview as a substance with physical properties, highlighting the unpredictable nature of history-taking in authentic contexts and the need to adapt accordingly.

By far the most common concept to which the students' metaphorical expressions related was that of progression along a path or track. This is not surprising, since the metaphor of a journey is one of the most common employed by speakers of English (Kövecses, 2010). However, in this case the expressions related to a specific type of journey: one that was expected to follow a pre-determined path. Such expressions implied that when patients told stories that students considered irrelevant, this was seen as a departure from the right path.

Susan told me: 'They go off the track all the time', and confided that she had learnt 'you can go off on that track, but just remember to come back later'. Walid found that 'sometimes the patients just jump off and suddenly start to talk about their past history'. Ashanka took a similar line to Andrew, saying she would let them talk, 'but when they've finished, I try to move it back to where I want it to be'. I became curious to know how they would respond when they noticed patients digressing in this way. Walid said: 'If they jump off a lot, talk about something not relevant, I just intercept them'. Jack says he's found that: 'You've got to learn to interrupt patients and just direct them to where you want to go'. But he implied disapproval when he described the tactics he had seen employed by some doctors: 'Some people are very abrupt and just plough straight on through'.

Employing this metaphor when talking about medical interviews implies a belief that, ideally, they should lead directly to a diagnosis. However, it obscures the relational functions of clinical interactions, including building trust and rapport, exploring a patient's experience of the illness, and identity construction. The same metaphorical expression has been applied to cognitive behaviour therapy sessions (Antaki & Jahoda, 2010). Therapists spoke about keeping a session on track, meaning keeping the patient focused on what the therapist saw as the main task of the interaction. They employed various strategies when they perceived that the patient was diverging from the track. This highlights a tension between the client's expectation that their concerns will be addressed, and the therapist's view about what should be accomplished within a particular session.

In a previous study, metaphorical expressions used by patients, students and clinical educators were analysed to explore how they conceptualised clinical relationships (Rees et al., 2007). Conceptual metaphors commonly used, including *war*, *hierarchy* and *the market*, characterised these relationships as adversarial. In my study, I found that for students talking about their encounters with patients, the track metaphor was dominant. As with the psychotherapists' study (Antaki & Jahoda, 2010), the tension between the path considered ideal by the student and the digressive course followed by many patients can be interpreted as an expression of divergent priorities. It evokes a sense of conflict or struggle, resonating with the findings of Rees et al. (2007). A more explicitly adversarial view of encounters between patients and medical students emerges from the analysis of stories in Chapter 6 of this book.

The precession of simulacra

The metaphors students use to describe their encounters with real patients suggest potential unintended consequences of extensive early exposure to simulated interactions. For example, it can lead students to see interactions with simulated patients as more authentic than those with real ones. Baudrillard's concept of the *precession of simulacra* (Baudrillard, 1994 [1981], p. 91) has been used to explore this idea (Bleakley & Bligh, 2009; Bligh & Bleakley, 2006). A simulacrum is a superficial likeness: a copy of a copy; or a copy 'where the original has been lost or never existed' (Bligh & Bleakley, 2006, p. 606). The term *precession* refers to situations in which a simulacrum precedes contact with the corresponding authentic object. Baudrillard explains the concept through an allegorical story about a map which becomes familiar to a traveller before he encounters the territory it represents. Something seems to be wrong with the country when it does not conform to the expectations conjured by his knowledge of the map. In other words, the traveller's perception of the territory is shaped, and potentially distorted, by the precession of the simulacrum: in this case, the map (Baudrillard, 1994 [1981]).

During my fieldwork, some tutors' advice to students leading up to their end-of-year examinations can be understood as an instance of the precession of simulacra.

The students' competence in clinical skills was evaluated by clinical teachers during their first clinical year through observation of their performance taking a history or carrying out an examination on a series of real patients. Many students chose patients for these assessments who presented more like simulated patients, in that they were more predictable than many real patients. At the end of the year they were assessed through Objective Structured Clinical Examinations (OSCEs), which commonly involved simulated patients.

During the OSCE, students were required to perform either a focused phys-ical examination or take a history about a specific problem and answer sub-sequent questions. They had to do this for a series of clinical scenarios, each within an eight-minute time limit. The patients in the exam could be actors with a script, or genuine patients with specific instructions as to what to do and say. The aim was for every candidate to be faced with the same tasks, enabling an equitable, standardised assessment of their competence (Levine & Swarz, 2008). The use of standardised or simulated patients in medical education is ubiquitous; however, the limitations and potential adverse consequences of this approach should be acknowledged.

Students may encounter difficulties in transferring to the real world the knowledge about clinical interactions they develop in simulated environments. Several authors have explored this idea in the literature (Bleakley & Bligh, 2008; Bligh & Bleakley, 2006; Hanna & Fins, 2006; Hatala, Marr, Cuncic, & Bacchus, 2011; Hodges, 2003; Huntley, Salmon, Fisher, Fletcher, & Young, 2012). Although many students find simulated experiences useful, there is a danger that some students will *simulate* learning – feign knowledge they do not have – in order to pass a test or exam. Alternatively, they may *dis-simulate* – conceal bad habits or negative attitudes they believe would nega-tively affect their assessment if revealed (Bligh & Bleakley, 2006; Hanna & Fins, 2006).

When I was interviewing students as their end-of-year exams approached, a number of them told me their tutors had advised them to stop practising on real patients and instead rehearse history and examination technique with their peers. Surprised, I asked Natalie, one of the students, why she thought they were given this advice.

It's because OSCE patients, they usually come in and have been prepped with a script and know – they've got one condition they've come in with, and they're good historians and they know exactly how long they've had this sort of pain and exactly where it started and that sort of thing. But real patients, they're – it's such a different art, because you're trying to manage people who have interesting social skills and people who want to talk about all their grandchildren and would just talk to you for hours and hours; so you're trying to keep directing them back to your questions and – it's very … like, with OSCE you've got eight minutes and it's much easier to do it on someone who knows what you're looking for.

It is understandable that the nature of assessment tasks drives students' learning, and that they will prepare in the way most likely to maximise their grades. It is also sensible that as novices, they are given more straightforward problems. But it does seem counter-productive if the assessment is designed in a way that preferentially tests how well they can interact with simulated, as opposed to authentic, patients. Another issue is that the short duration of each OSCE station tends to limit the focus in most cases to a single body system whereas in real life, sick people commonly present with multiple inter-related problems. As Natalie says, real patients tend to be complex and unpredictable. This way of relating to patients has the potential to influence students' emerging identities. A story told by another student named Ashanka provides a further opportunity to explore this issue.

Struggle for an integrated identity

I don't know how to cut them off!

During my fieldwork, I heard about the struggles many students experience when they start learning in the hospital. At the time of this interview, Ashanka and I have met a few times and I have attended some of her bedside tutorials. From our conversations, she knows I am a novice researcher and a senior doctor with daughters about her age. Our interview takes place in a tutorial room far from the bustle of the wards and clinics, but announcements over the public-address system remind us we are still in the hospital. About halfway through the interview, I comment that some research suggests medical students' capacity for empathy can diminish during their time in the medical course. Her response indicates that this observation resonates with her experience. In her story, she associates reported problems of empathy decline with the way students are taught to respond to patients' stories.

> I can see that happening. I remember I was, like, taking a history from a patient with my tutor there and, like, after it was over he's, like: [Speaks in an authoritative tone] 'You need to learn how to cut patients off, 'cause otherwise you're not going to get information from them'.
>
> [Speaks loudly] And – I don't know how to cut them off, because they have to tell me things and to them it's important! I know, to the history it's not, but to them it is! But you know, my tutor was saying, 'If you're taking physician exams you have five minutes to get a history, you can't afford to let a patient blather on, you need to just tell them: "OK, and moving on – this, this, this, this and this"'. [Slaps her hand on the table each time she says the word 'this'.]
>
> [Speaks more quietly] A lot of it just seems to be learning how to interrupt a patient quite gently, and moving it on to, I suppose, paths that you'd like the

conversation to take; but ... at the same time, I feel like you miss out on a lot if you do that.

OK, yeah, so time's a big issue. And that's part of the reason –

Time is the big issue. Yeah, we're pretty much taught to –

[Emergency announcement over the public-address system]: Attention please! Metcall, Ward 4 South; Metcall, Ward 4 South.

– act like that, I guess.

To cut them off?

Yes. Because you don't have time and you need to get a good history if you want to treat a patient well.

A multi-vocal narrative

One of the striking things about this story is that Ashanka speaks with multiple voices. Initially, I feel as though I'm listening to an adolescent talking, because she speaks informally, liberally sprinkling her sentences with the word 'like'. She adopts a more authoritative tone when she speaks as the tutor. Her portrayal

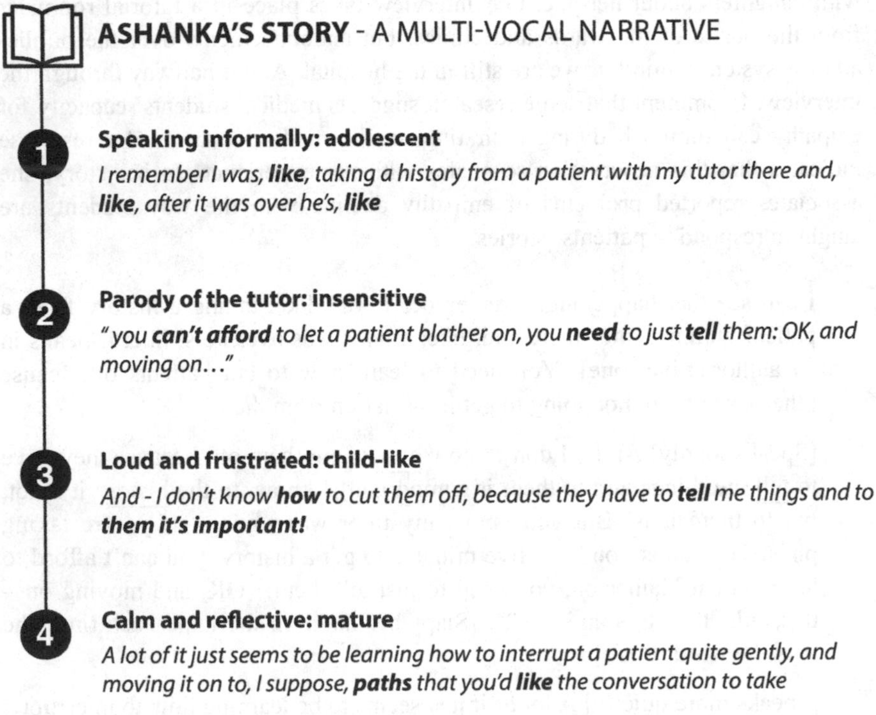

ASHANKA'S STORY - A MULTI-VOCAL NARRATIVE

1

Speaking informally: adolescent

*I remember I was, **like**, taking a history from a patient with my tutor there and, **like**, after it was over he's, **like***

2

Parody of the tutor: insensitive

*" you **can't afford** to let a patient blather on, you **need** to just **tell** them: OK, and moving on..."*

3

Loud and frustrated: child-like

*And - I don't know **how** to cut them off, because they have to **tell** me things and to them it's important!*

4

Calm and reflective: mature

*A lot of it just seems to be learning how to interrupt a patient quite gently, and moving it on to, I suppose, **paths** that you'd **like** the conversation to take*

Figure 3.1 Ashanka's story: a multi-vocal narrative.

suggests exaggeration or parody, although it is impossible to be certain exactly what he actually said and how. Then she becomes agitated and speaks more loudly, as she wrestles with the competing demands of the situation, and it seems as though she is speaking as a child, appealing to me to resolve her dilemma. Finally, she is calmer and more reflective, representing herself as more sensitive than the tutor and more mature than the way she had previously represented herself.

The way Ashanka represents the tutor's speech implies he has a dismissive attitude towards patients' stories; she associates this with the reports of a decline in empathy during medical school. Although she acknowledges the need for key facts about the illness to be gleaned within time constraints, she says this can be done 'quite gently' rather than 'cutting off' the patient's story. In doing so, she identifies herself as someone who is trying to find her own, more respectful way of relating to patients, instead of uncritically following her tutor's directions.

Ashanka's story confirms the multiple and dynamic nature of identity and reveals the struggle between the values and practices associated with her established identities, and those expected of her emerging identities. Although she starts off presenting her view as being in opposition to that of the tutor, Ashanka moderates her position as she acknowledges the problem of time, speaking of gently leading patients back to the path. This is an active, creative process that results in the emergence of a new professional identity and its integration with established identities. It is not simply a matter of imitating or passively absorbing the values and cultural practices of the profession.

The story does identity work because it is a vehicle for Ashanka to construct and perform identities using multiple voices, which are juxtaposed with one another. When she speaks with the voice of the tutor, she conveys her interpretation of his position, and also her negative evaluation of his attitude; but this is expressed indirectly, using the narrative device of ventriloquation – speaking through his words (Bakhtin, 1981; Reissman, 2008; Wortham, 2001). In this case, she renders his speech as parody, and juxtaposes it with the parts of the story told in the other voices.

While the tutor dismisses the patient's tangential discourse as being of no consequence, Ashanka's opening statement links the neglect of patients' stories to a purported decline in students' capacity for empathy. Her telling of the story in this context implies that she believes the tutor's capacity to empathise with patients is diminished. This is reinforced by her later comment that students are taught to respond in this way. This is an example of *emergence*: meanings which arise from events that take place both before and after the narrative itself (Wortham, 2001).

Interactional positioning

Ashanka constructs and performs identities by using multiple voices and positioning herself in relation to her interviewer and story characters. This offers insight into the relationship between her multiple identities (Monrouxe, 2010).

She initially positions herself closer to patients and more distant from the tutor. At one point, she also positions herself in relation to me, someone much older with considerable clinical experience, in rather a child-like way. Loudly expressing her frustration at the conflicting demands upon her, she seems to be appealing for understanding or advice. She later adopts a more mature, considered voice as she reflects on how these competing priorities might be resolved. This shift in voice during an autobiographical narrative performance shows how the narrator's identity is performed and negotiated within a storytelling event (Wortham, 2001).

Rather than uncritically complying with her tutor's instructions, Ashanka struggles to reconcile the conflicting demands of the situation. There is a clash between the behaviour expected of her as a medical student, and that which she has previously valued as a respectful person. With the words 'quite gently', she indicates that she is seeking a way of working with patients as a doctor that would be harmonious with her established identities. This illustrates that medical students' professional identity formation is an active process and shows how emerging identities can be integrated with those that are more established (Holmes, Jenks, & Stonington, 2011; Goldie, 2012; Monrouxe, 2010).

The degree of integration between an individual's multiple identities has a bearing on the diversity of other people with whom they can identify (Monrouxe, 2010; Roccas & Brewer, 2002). The construction and integration of an emerging professional identity into a person's established identities should be acknowledged as a fundamental component of medical education (Goldie, 2012). It is likely that students who are able to identify with a greater variety of people will have a greater capacity to empathise with patients (Monrouxe, 2010).

Medical students reflecting on their encounters with patients often believe that developing a medical student identity requires them to give up their ability to adopt a layperson's perspective (Yardley, Brosnan, & Richardson, 2013). They described feeling compelled to hide their true opinions or to express inconsistent views when speaking with different groups of people. This indicates that for the person concerned, their emerging identities are compartmentalised from established identities, rather than being integrated with them (Monrouxe, 2010; Roccas, Sagiv, Schwartz, Halevy, & Eidelson, 2008).

Identity work at the bedside

There's no-one else like me!

Just like students, patients use stories to construct and perform their identities, even when little attention is paid to their efforts. Next, I analyse how one patient accomplishes this during a bedside teaching encounter as he engages with a medical student in a collaborative process of storytelling, watched by fellow students, their tutor and me.

> I'm waiting with a group of medical students and their tutor Robert outside the door of a patient's single room on the coronary care unit. Jack, one of the

students, has interviewed him the previous day, and asks if he would mind another student having a chat with him. He replies, 'No, that's OK. Go for it'. As the rest of the group files in slowly, he says: 'Come on in; I won't bite!'

Mr Hartmann is a fit-looking elderly man sitting up on his elevated bed in a relaxed pose, leaning back on the pillows and grasping his right leg below the knee. Multi-coloured ECG leads protrude from the pocket of his pyjama top. On the end of the bed sit two large blue plastic bags containing his clothing, suggesting that he may soon be discharged home or transferred to another ward. He points towards Jack and addresses the rest of the group. 'He did the lot the other day. Very thorough, he was'.

After a brief debate, it's agreed that Anna will take the history. She introduces herself and begins. 'Can you tell me what brought you to hospital?'

'I came in with atrial fibrillation', he replies.

'OK, so what symptoms did you have?'

'I had a feeling of tightness in my chest, like emphysema. It built up over three or four days. First, it was like a flutter in my chest. Next day, that was Tuesday, it lasted for longer. I said to myself, 'There's something wrong somewhere'. The following day, Wednesday, I had to stop. I called an ambulance'.

'So, did it come on gradually, then?'

'It wasn't hard, like an asthma attack. It sort of crept up on me'.

'And did you have any pain?' Anna probes further into his symptoms.

'No pain, just a sort of pressure … like being crushed'.

'And was your heart racing?'

'Yes, it was'.

'And was your heartbeat regular?'

'No, it misses a beat. Actually, it's been irregular since I was very young. I used to get asthma badly. When I was a baby, I was clinically dead twice. When I was born, I only weighed two pounds. That was in 1935, in a bush hospital. Times were hard in those days. They didn't have any humidicribs'.

'And is your asthma better now?'

'Nothing like as bad as it used to be, since I got the puffers. I get short of breath and tightness. Ventolin helps a bit. I puff and I snort, and I carry on!' He laughs at his own description of an asthma attack, and the audience joins in.

'So, what tests have you had since you came in?'

'I had the angios – that showed they couldn't put a stent in. The blockage was on the cusp of two veins, so they couldn't do the angiogram'.

'What treatment have you had for the heart problem?'

'Well, I had to start on warfarin'.

'So, have you ever had any strokes?'

[Pause] 'Well, I'm not sure. I was in bed once; the wife was listening to the radio. I got a funny feeling. I said to her, 'Why'd you turn the light out?' and she said, 'I didn't turn the light out'. Turns out, my left eye had shut down. So, they sent me to the hospital, and they said I'd had a clot to the left eye. The doctors injected dye in my eye, and I asked, 'Can I have a look?' I could see all the veins outlined in red. I enjoyed seeing the lovely students – like yourselves. [Smiles and looks at group] I explained all this to them'.

'They would have loved you. [warmly] Have you ever had any clots in the legs?'

'No – but sometimes they call me a clot!' The students join in his laughter as he makes a joke at his own expense.

'And you've had asthma – and emphysema as well?'

'Yes, I got emphysema later on, from smoking. I smoked from age 13 till I was about 48. I used to smoke up to 100 a day. I worked a 22-hour day, doing a security job, while I was starting my own business. I couldn't afford it now!'

'Does anyone in your family have a history of similar problems?'

'No, there's nobody else like me!' [Smiling] As we prepare to leave, he adds earnestly: 'It's a very serious thing you people are doing. The doctors here are the best in Melbourne. You'll learn a lot from them'. We thank him, wish him well and file out to gather in a tutorial room where Anna presents the case to Robert.

'Mr Hartmann is a 76-year-old man admitted with atrial fibrillation five days ago, after several days of irregular palpitations. He has a history of past heavy smoking, asthma and emphysema and a retinal thrombosis. He has had a coronary angiogram and is now on medical treatment, including warfarin'.

Robert gives Anna feedback about her history-taking efforts and discusses treatment. Before moving on, he declares: 'He is a stock-standard patient'.

Stories within stories

Figure 3.2 is a visual representation of the relationship between the storytelling events and narrated events in this excerpt, and the people involved. The stories about Mr Hartmann's life – the narrated events – are told within the storytelling event of the tutorial. This book is another storytelling event, in which the story about the tutorial is told. The main focus of the analysis is the storytelling event of

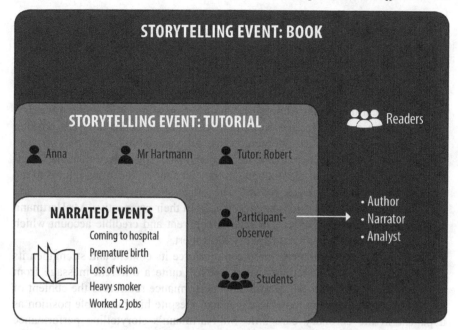

Figure 3.2 Mr Hartmann's story: multi-level analysis.

the tutorial, containing the narrated events; the people present at the tutorial are part of the narrative context. Multiple researcher identities are shown spanning the two storytelling events. As participant-observer, while I watch and take notes, I join in the laughter at Mr Hartmann's jokes and thank him as we depart. From time to time, we meet each other's gaze as I stand at the foot of his bed. I am the narrator of this reconstructed story, and also the narrative analyst and author of this book.

I have used the speakers' words as closely as possible, but this is a reconstruction of the interaction rather than a faithful reproduction, because I recorded it with hand-written notes. As the narrator, I describe elements of the context that are not evident from the speakers' words, such as the position of people in the room, their mode of dress, age group or demeanour. As narrative analyst I carry out the steps of the analytic process, and as the author I report on them. Enacting multiple identities requires me to adopt several perspectives on the story, expanding the interpretations arising from the research. This diagram was inspired by those used by Wortham (2000) in his work on interactional positioning, but his diagrams are used for a different purpose: to show how words or phrases from the narrated events are associated with certain types of speakers.

Analysis and interpretation

Information about the context in which a story was told often provides clues as to why it was told in a particular way (Gubrium & Holstein, 2009; Wortham, 2001). Before we entered his room, Jack asked Mr Hartmann whether he would be happy for another student to have a chat with him. The framing of the encounter as an informal conversation may have facilitated his garrulous style of storytelling, and their earlier positive interaction may have contributed to his relaxed and confident demeanour.

During the interview, Anna collaborates with Mr Hartmann, steering a course between paying attention to his stories and gathering the information she needs to make a medical diagnosis. Although each of her questions is oriented towards a specific response, he seizes the opportunity to elaborate on his answers, offering autobiographical anecdotes. She neither interrupts nor invites him to expand on them, unless events seem relevant to his diagnosis. The power dynamics shift back and forth throughout the dialogue as they take turns, and Anna returns to the medical history after each anecdote. The other students' close attention and laughter at his humorous asides suggest that from their perspective, Mr Hartmann is an accomplished storyteller. He gives a coherent and credible account which enables Anna to construct a case history for Robert.

The way a narrative is performed can reinforce its content and strengthen its rhetorical power, but sometimes it can convey quite a different message from what is said. In this case, Mr Hartmann's performance reinforces the content of his stories, apart from one notable exception. Despite his vulnerable position as a patient in the coronary care unit, Mr Hartmann's storytelling performance identifies him as resilient, strong and assertive. The raised position of his bed evokes a theatre stage, placing him at the same level as the audience. This, along with his relaxed posture, gives the impression that he considers his status equal with theirs. His air of confidence is reinforced when he tells the students: 'I won't bite', implying that they seem hesitant and in need of reassurance. The props or significant objects that are part of the narrative context also contribute to his performance. In this case, the large blue plastic bags containing his belongings suggest that he is about to be discharged from the coronary care unit.

Mr Hartmann employs self-deprecating humour throughout the interaction, and this seems to influence his audience's responses to his stories. The tales of his premature birth and ill health could have aroused pity, but the way he tells them seems to evoke appreciation for his resilience. A potential consequence is that any negative emotions provoked by his present illness, such as fear, anger or frustration, are hidden. This is a notable omission, although it may be related to the tutorial setting, as he might not be comfortable discussing these emotions with students. However, in his closing remarks he speaks earnestly, casting aside his jocular tone as he reminds students of the serious business they are engaged in. By referring to the importance of what they are learning, he could be implicitly acknowledging a degree of vulnerability.

The acknowledgement and exploration of negative emotional cues and concerns has been shown to be beneficial for patients (Zimmerman & Del Piccolo, 2007). However, their expression in medical consultations tends to be infrequent and subtle (Mjaaland, Finset, Jensen, & Gulbrandsen, 2011). Physicians often implicitly discourage the disclosure of concerns and when they are expressed, may fail to grasp their importance (Zimmerman & Del Piccolo, 2007). A sensitive listener, noting Mr Hartmann's change in tone, might return later to offer him a more private opportunity to discuss this aspect of his illness experience.

The stories Mr Hartmann chooses to tell share a common thread: he survived his premature birth against the odds, smoked heavily while working long hours at two jobs and delayed several days before presenting to hospital with his racing heartbeat. These stories indicate that he identifies himself as a strong and resilient man. Mr Hartmann performs his identity in this way while acknowledging the link between smoking and his health problems. The stories place the present illness in the context of his life, creating a degree of coherence which can be an important function of storytelling (Garro & Mattingly, 2000).

Heteroglossia, answerability and intertextuality

Bakhtin coined the term *heteroglossia*, referring to the idea that the multiple *voices* used by a speaker within a given story contribute to its meaning (Holquist, 2002). Like Ashanka, Mr Hartmann speaks with many voices as he collaboratively constructs and performs this story. By appropriating medical language and weaving it into *his* story, he speaks with the voice of medicine, identifies himself in relation to the students as a teacher and potentially elevates his status by association (Gubrium & Holstein, 2009). His amusing anecdotes identify him as a joker, and when he refers playfully to the students in his eye hospital story as: 'lovely ... like yourselves', Anna responds in a similar vein: 'They would have loved you'.

Bakhtin argued that communicative acts should not be considered in isolation, because: 'any utterance is a link in the chain of speech communion' (Bakhtin, 1986, p. 84). While Anna collaborates with Mr Hartmann to produce the story, she is aware that she will be required to retell it in the genre of the case presentation. This knowledge would influence her contributions to the storytelling event of the tutorial and the way she collaborates in its telling. As a result, the story yet to be told to the tutor influences the story being constructed in the present moment between herself and Mr Hartmann (Gubrium & Holstein, 2009). In any dialogue, 'forming itself in an atmosphere of the already spoken, the word is at the same time determined by that which has not yet been said but which is ... anticipated by the answering word' (Bakhtin, 1981, p. 280). Bakhtin used the term *answerability* to describe this essential property of both spoken and written communication.

This story contains many examples of intertextuality as well, as Mr Hartmann includes words, ideas and plots from other stories into new tales about his experience. They include accounts he must have heard from other people, for example, about his premature birth and why he could not have a stent inserted. Elements from other stories are not simply replicated by narrators, but are used to construct new ones, and the way narrators do this contributes to their identity work (Frank, 2010; Wortham, 2001). Bakhtin argued that the word 'becomes one's own only when the speaker populates it ... with his own accent, when he appropriates the word, adapting it to his own ... intention' (Bakhtin, 1981, p. 293).

Parallel narratives of disease, illness and identity

Through this analysis, distinct threads can be discerned, which are represented visually in Figure 3.3. Each of Anna's questions, posed with the intention of seeking diagnostic information (first column from the left) results in responses that can be categorised into two groups. The first group relates to Mr Hartmann's medical diagnosis and treatment (second column from left) and the second to the illness in the context of his life (third column). Combined with his storytelling performance, these sets of responses contribute to the construction of multiple identities, represented in the column on the right.

Mr Hartmann declares in response to a question about his family history, that: 'There's nobody else like me!' Although this may appear to be a facetious aside, it can also be read in this context as an assertion that he is a unique individual. Despite having gathered considerable information about his life, including the way he manages his health and responds to illness, Anna presents a story to Robert that is stripped of colour and richness. Through explicit teaching and by observing others' presentations, she has learnt the style and content expected when a student presents a patient's story as a clinical case (Anspach, 1998; Donnelly, 1997). Anna may well have formed an impression about the kind of person Mr Hartmann is, and the potential impact this might have on his relationships with doctors. However, this knowledge is not considered worthy of mention in the presentation.

There is a stark contrast between Mr Hartmann's view of himself as an individual and Robert's characterisation of him as a 'stock-standard' or typical patient. His statement is intended to impress on students the important fact that the pattern of Mr Hartmann's story resembles that of many others with the same condition. Unfortunately, he fails to also acknowledge the relevance of individual characteristics to the management of the patient, including the nature of the therapeutic relationship and the way options may be negotiated. It is possible that in his own practice, Robert does take into account knowledge gained from patients' stories. However, his idea of the clinical teaching role does not encompass this level of reflection. Anna's interaction with Mr Hartmann displays considerable skill, given her novice status, but this is not considered worthy of mention. During my fieldwork, I rarely heard a tutor congratulate a student for navigating a successful path through a patient's complex stories.

Identity and academic learning

Research in other settings has demonstrated that identity construction and academic learning are inextricably connected (Wortham, 2006). As mentioned earlier, students' early learning about how to interact with patients is mediated, involving the use of texts, lectures or simplified role-playing scenarios. The use of simulated encounters to teach and assess communication skills is widespread and perceived as safe, simple and consistent. However, its exclusive use before students encounter real patients may have unintended consequences and potentially shape students' emerging identities (Bligh & Bleakley, 2006). Students

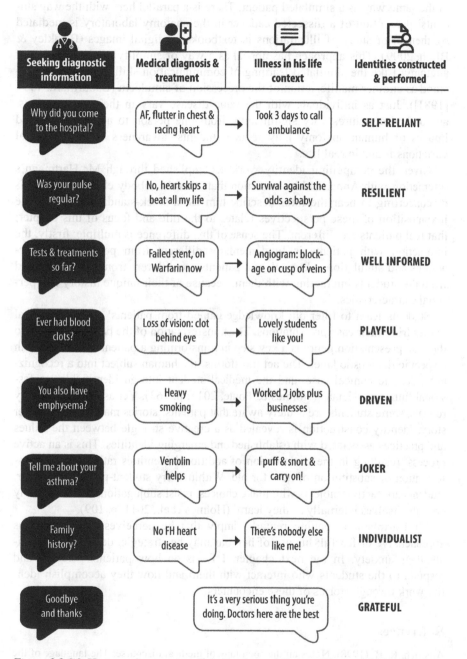

Seeking diagnostic information	Medical diagnosis & treatment	Illness in his life context	Identities constructed & performed
Why did you come to the hospital?	AF, flutter in chest & racing heart →	Took 3 days to call ambulance	**SELF-RELIANT**
Was your pulse regular?	No, heart skips a beat all my life →	Survival against the odds as baby	**RESILIENT**
Tests & treatments so far?	Failed stent, on Warfarin now →	Angiogram: block-age on cusp of veins	**WELL INFORMED**
Ever had blood clots?	Loss of vision: clot behind eye →	Lovely students like you!	**PLAYFUL**
You also have emphysema?	Heavy smoking →	Worked 2 jobs plus businesses	**DRIVEN**
Tell me about your asthma?	Ventolin helps →	I puff & snort & carry on!	**JOKER**
Family history?	No FH heart disease →	There's nobody else like me!	**INDIVIDUALIST**
Goodbye and thanks		It's a very serious thing you're doing. Doctors here are the best	**GRATEFUL**

Figure 3.3 Mr Hartmann's story: parallel narratives of disease, illness and identity.

may perceive real patients as less authentic because they expect them to interact in the same way as a simulated patient. There is a parallel here with the way students' perception of a dissected cadaver in the anatomy laboratory is mediated by their prior study of illustrations in textbooks or digital images (Bleakley & Bligh, 2009). This approach has appeal as a way of simplifying the learning of anatomy. Like the simulated learning of communication skills, it can be understood as another manifestation of the precession of simulacra (Baudrillard, 1994 [1981]). Just as individuals with the same disease vary in their presentations, anatomical structures vary significantly from one person to another. Idealised images of human anatomy may reduce students' awareness of the structural variations found in real life.

Given the compelling identity work accomplished through Mr Hartmann's interaction with Anna, and his assertion that 'there's nobody else like me', it is disconcerting to hear the tutor describe him as 'a stock-standard patient'. The juxtaposition of these perspectives relates to the title and focus of this chapter: that real patients are different. The sense of this difference is multiple: firstly, the interaction with patients is fundamentally different from peer-to-peer interactions and simulations. As well, real patients are different from each other, and from the students interacting with them, because of their unique history and personal characteristics.

Students learn to filter out knowledge gained from patients' autobiographical stories from their case presentations. The transformation of the patient's story into the case presentation genre is a key step in transforming a patient into a case with a specific diagnostic label. The act transforms 'the human subject into a recognizable, generic clinical case, and the medical student into an identifiable, professional future physician' (Holmes & Ponte, 2011, p. 163). Yet as Ashanka's story reveals, some students are acutely aware that patients' stories matter. Through her story, identity construction is revealed as a creative struggle between the values and practices associated with established and emerging identities. This is an active process, resulting in the construction of additional identities rather than a transformation or substitution of new for old. Within every student-patient encounter, students are 'active subjects who make choices, resist subjugation, and ... actively craft themselves internally as they learn' (Holmes et al., 2011, p. 109).

Mr Hartmann's opening remarks imply that he perceives the students as apprehensive or fearful; his use of humour may be strategic, designed to alleviate their anxiety. In the next chapter, I focus on how patients perceive and respond to the students who interact with them and how they accomplish identity work through stories of these encounters.

References

Anspach, R. R. (1998). Notes on the sociology of medical discourse: The language of the case presentation. *Journal of Health and Social Behaviour, 29*(4), 357–375.

Antaki, C., & Jahoda, A. (2010). Psychotherapists' practices in keeping a session 'on-track' in the face of clients' 'off-track' talk. *Communication and Medicine, 7*(1), 11–21.

Bakhtin, M. M. (1981). Discourse in the novel (C. Emerson & M. Holquist, Trans.). In M. Holquist (Ed.), *The dialogic imagination* (pp. 59–422). Austin, TX: University of Texas Press.

Bakhtin, M. M. (1986). The problem of speech genres (V. W. McGee, Trans.). In C. Emerson & M. Holquist (Eds.), *Speech genres and other late essays* (pp. 60–102). Austin, TX: University of Texas Press.

Baudrillard, J. (1994 [1981]). *Simulacra and simulation* (S. F. Glaser, Trans.). Ann Arbor, MI: University of Michigan Press.

Bleakley, A., & Bligh, J. (2008). Students learning from patients: Let's get real in medical education. *Advances in Health Sciences Education, 13,* 89–107.

Bleakley, A., & Bligh, J. (2009). Who can resist Foucault? *Journal of Medicine & Philosophy, 34*(4), 368–383.

Bligh, J., & Bleakley, A. (2006). Distributing menus to hungry learners: Can learning by simulation become simulation of learning? *Medical Teacher, 28*(7), 606–613. doi:10.1080/01421590601042335

Donnelly, W. J. (1997). The language of medical case histories. *Annals of Internal Medicine, 127*(11), 1045–1048.

Frank, A. W. (2010). *Letting stories breathe: A socio-narratology.* Chicago, IL & London: University of Chicago Press.

Garro, L. C., & Mattingly, C. (2000). Narrative as construct and construction. In C. Mattingly & L. C. Garro (Eds.), *Narrative and the cultural construction of illness and healing* (pp. 1–49). Berkeley, CA: University of California Press.

Goldie, J. (2012). The formation of professional identity in medical students: Considerations for educators. *Medical Teacher, 34,* e641–e648.

Gubrium, J. F., & Holstein, J. A. (2009). *Analyzing narrative reality.* Los Angeles, CA: Sage.

Hanna, M., & Fins, J. J. (2006). Viewpoint: Power and communication: Why simulation training ought to be complemented by experiential and humanist learning. *Academic Medicine, 81*(3), 265–270.

Hatala, R., Marr, S., Cuncic, C., & Bacchus, C. M. (2011). Modification of an OSCE format to enhance patient continuity in a high-stakes assessment of clinical performance. *BMC Medical Education, 11*(23), 1–5.

Hodges, B. (2003). OSCE! Variations on a theme by Harden. *Medical Education, 37,* 1134–1140.

Holmes, S., Jenks, A., & Stonington, S. (2011). Clinical subjectivation: Anthropologies of contemporary biomedical training. *Culture, Medicine and Psychiatry, 35,* 105–112. doi:10.1007/s11013-011-9207-1

Holmes, S., & Ponte, M. (2011). En-case-ing the patient: Disciplining uncertainty in medical student patient presentations. *Culture, Medicine and Psychiatry, 35,* 163–182. doi:10.1007/s11013-011-9213-3

Holquist, M. (2002). *Dialogism* (2nd ed.). London & New York: Routledge.

Huntley, C., Salmon, P., Fisher, P., Fletcher, I., & Young, B. (2012). LUCAS: A theoretically informed instrument to assess clinical communication in objective structured clinical examinations. *Medical Education, 46,* 267–276. doi:10.1111/j.1365-2923. 2011.04162.x

Kövecses, Z. (2010). *Metaphor: A practical introduction* (2nd ed.). New York: Oxford University Press.

Lakoff, G., & Johnson, M. (1980). *Metaphors we live by.* Chicago, IL & London: The University of Chicago Press.

Levine, A., & Swarz, M. (2008). Standardized patients: The 'other' simulation. *Journal of Critical Care, 23*(2), 179–184.

Mjaaland, T. A., Finset, A., Jensen, B. F., & Gulbrandsen, P. (2011). Patients' negative emotional cues and concerns in hospital consultations: A video-based observational study. *Patient Education and Counselling, 85*, 356–362. doi:10.1016/j.pec/2010.12.031

Monrouxe, L. (2010). Identity, identification and medical education: Why should we care? *Medical Education, 44*(1), 40–49. doi:10.1111/j.1365-2923.2009.03440.x

Rees, C., Knight, L., & Wilkinson, C. (2007). Doctors being up there and we being down there: A metaphorical analysis of talk about student/doctor relationships. *Social Science and Medicine, 65*, 725–737.

Reissman, C. K. (2008). *Narrative methods for the human sciences.* Los Angeles, CA: Sage.

Roccas, S., & Brewer, M. B. (2002). Social identity complexity. *Personality and Social Psychology Review, 6*(2), 88–106. doi:10.1207/s15327957pspr0602_01

Roccas, S., Sagiv, L., Schwartz, S., Halevy, N., & Eidelson, R. (2008). Toward a unifying model of identification with groups: Integrating theoretical perspectives. *Personality and Social Psychology Review, 12*(3), 280–306. doi:10.1177/1088868308319225

Salmon, P., & Young, B. (2011). Creativity in clinical communication: From communication skills to skilled communication. *Medical Education, 45*, 217–226.

Wortham, S. (2000). Interactional positioning and narrative self-construction. *Narrative Inquiry, 10*(1), 157–184. doi:10.1075/ni.10.1.11wor

Wortham, S. (2001). *Narratives in action: A strategy for research and analysis.* New York: Teachers College Press.

Wortham, S. (2006). *Learning identity: The joint emergence of social identification and academic learning.* New York: Cambridge University Press.

Yardley, S., Brosnan, C., & Richardson, J. (2013). The consequences of authentic early experience for medical students: Creation of mētis. *Medical Education, 47*(1), 109–119. doi:10.1111/j.1365-2923.2012.04287.x

Zimmerman, C., & Del Piccolo, L. (2007). Cues and concerns by patients in medical consultations: A literature review. *Psychological Bulletin, 133*(3), 438–463.

4   Imagining the students' world

> Well, I think it's up to me; because they are who they are and, you know, to a
> certain extent naïve and unsophisticated, it's my duty to make it as easy as
> possible for them. Because it would be embarrassing, and I can see the other
> side of the coin. ... If I think they're very embarrassed altogether, I pretend
> not to notice them at all. If I think they're up to it, well then, I'll have a little
> 'to-and-fro' there.
>
> Rita, a patient in the medical ward

Engaging with patients' stories

In this chapter, I turn to stories told by patients that reveal their interpretations of
the character, motivation or emotional state of students they have encountered.
These stories highlight the relational nature of identities constructed by patients
when talking about their interactions with students. Rita portrays some of the
medical students she has met as naïve and embarrassed. She feels compassion
towards them and acts to alleviate their discomfort, but her response depends on
how uneasy they appear. She will often engage in a little banter with them, but
only if they don't seem too anxious. Rita constructs and performs an identity for
herself in relation to the students as she tells this story during the research interview. By characterising the students as naïve, anxious and embarrassed, she
identifies herself in relation to them as sophisticated, relaxed and confident.

Much of the research into health care encounters focuses on the instrumental
skills and techniques of communication. However, the *relational* aspects of these
interactions are often of greater importance to patients (Goldie, 2012; Salmon &
Young, 2011). Patient perspectives on medical students' subjective experience
have received little attention in the medical education literature. However, there
are some studies addressing the meanings patients associate with their *own*
experiences in clinical teaching contexts (Chretien, Goldman, Craven, &
Faselis, 2010; Fletcher, Rankey, & Stern, 2005). This chapter confirms that
although many patients are willing participants, their involvement carries risks as
well as potential benefits. Explaining carefully to patients what they can expect
before proceeding with clinical teaching interactions and debriefing with them
afterwards can enhance the potential benefits and minimise risks (Chretien et al.,

2010; Fletcher, Furney, & Stern, 2007; Nair, Coughlan, & Hensley, 1997; Romano, 1941).

Writing about his experience of being treated for prostate cancer, the late author Anatole Broyard expressed a desire for his doctor to see him as a whole person (Frank, 2004). The radically different kind of clinical relationship he imagined involved him making an appraisal of his doctor, just as he himself was evaluated. He wrote: 'While he inevitably feels superior to me because he is the doctor and I am the patient, I'd like him to know that I feel superior to him too, that he is my patient also and I have my diagnosis of him' (Broyard, 1992, p. 45). Broyard highlights the usual disparity in status and agency between physician and patient, even as he turns it on its head.

In the same way, each of the patients whose stories are told in this chapter has their diagnosis of the students. They draw attention to the complex power relations that arise within clinical interactions, including the fact that power is sometimes contested in surprising ways. This illuminates the complex relationship between social status, power dynamics and identity construction. Power and knowledge have been shown to be inextricably linked to identity in school-based learning and this is also true for medical education in clinical settings (Wortham, 2006). Patients' stories reveal that they have the capacity to be active agents in students' learning, rather than merely the passive material on which they are taught.

The stories in this chapter highlight the need for models of clinical teaching based on active patient collaboration, so that student-patient interactions become sites for knowledge *production* rather than merely *reproduction* (Bleakley & Bligh, 2008). In other words, through unique clinical encounters, students and patients collaborate to generate new knowledge about an individual's experience, which provides insight into those of other people. At present there is a heavy reliance in the construction of professional identities on role modelling: the imitation of the behaviour of clinical teachers or other clinicians that learners admire. Another way of constructing identity is in relation to patients through an appreciation of difference (Bleakley & Bligh, 2008). Learning to recognise the difference between our own perceptions and priorities and those of another person can enhance our capacity for empathy (Bleakley & Bligh, 2008; Frank, 2002, 2004).

Peter and Harvey's stories are different in some ways but are similar in that they both accomplish substantial identity work. While carrying out the analysis, I became aware of important parallels between two kinds of storytelling events: the student-patient encounter and the research interview. Interactions between research participants and interviewers are important sites for identity work, with their associated creative struggles. My exploration of these parallel, interwoven events enhances the interpretation of each narrative, and demonstrates one of the valuable aspects of a dialogic approach.

Responding to students with empathy

During fieldwork, an ethnographer may encounter a turning point: a moment when something happens that unexpectedly alters the direction of the research

(Murchison, 2010). My interview with Peter was just such a moment. He was the first patient I interviewed for this study and as he spoke about his experiences with students, I realised that he had his diagnosis of them – just as Broyard did of his doctor (Broyard, 1992). I had not previously thought about how patients imagined students' experience, or how important this might be to their identity work. This was to influence the direction of the research and expand the scope of my investigation.

Unlike the other patient interviews, which were carried out in hospital, this one took place at Peter's home. I first met him during a tutorial, but he was discharged before I could arrange an interview. When I contacted him, he was enthusiastic about participating and invited me to visit his home. Peter had been transferred to the Hospital in the Home programme because he had a serious infection requiring several weeks of intravenous therapy, which was continued at home with visiting medical and nursing support daily.

We sat comfortably in Peter's lounge room, which was adjacent to the kitchen. As we spoke, we could hear his wife washing the dishes and, later, preparing a meal. Although she did not participate actively, her presence was evident through the sounds of her work and she would have been able to hear our conversation. The short excerpts that follow were selected to illustrate how Peter constructed identity relationally through his characterisations of the students and his responses to them. After he told me how it had taken weeks in hospital and exhaustive tests for his fever and abdominal pain to be diagnosed, I asked him about his experiences with the students. Peter told me about an occasion when they came to see him in a small group, then another about a time when a student tried to insert an intravenous line.

The students approach

So, during the time that you were in hospital, did you see a lot of medical students?

Oh, there's quite a few come through, yes.

Did they come, like, when I saw you, we were with a tutorial group, but did they come on their own as well to see you?

There was a couple – er – that came in twos and p'raps threes.

They heard you were interesting.

Yes, sort of walked in and like – er – it was quite hilarious because – er – my kids, when they were growing up, did exactly the same thing when they wanted something: they stood around on one leg and said: [switches to a high-pitched, whining tone] 'Oh, would you mind?', you know. [I laugh at his performance]

So, the main thing for you, when they came on their own, was that it was funny, 'cause they wanted something from you.

Well you could tell, yeah.

By their body language?

That's right.

So – and when they did that, and they're sort of going 'Would you mind?', and standing on one leg, how did you react to that?

Oh, I didn't mind at all. A few of them were game to poke and prod, you know, feel, which was OK by me.

Yeah so – what was that like for you, being examined by them?

Oh, I didn't mind.

Did it – was it painful at all, or –?

Oh – [pause] if they hit the right spot it was a bit sore. [Interviewer laughs] I mean –

That didn't bother you too much, that they might hurt you?

Well no, they couldn't – I mean they couldn't really hurt me that bad. And – I mean the whole thing is that – they've gotta learn, haven't they?

The intravenous line

There was – a lass there doing – er – third year, whatever. And er – she was there – she was there for training. And she wanted to put the … line in the [indicates his right hand] – whatever you call it –

The intravenous line?

Intravenous line in the back of the hand. And of course, they'd had a few goes at – these were a bit sore, so they were trying to put it in up further, and – er – she had one go and was very embarrassed and couldn't get in. [Interviewer laughs]

So how did you feel about a student doing that?

And then – and had to hand it over to the nurse. And the nurse said: 'Well, you could go in there'. And then she said: 'Would you mind if' – I can't think of the girl's name – and I said, 'No, go ahead'. And anyway, she finally succeeded with a bit of help from the nurse.

Ok so – you were happy to kind of –

Oh, yeah. [Emphatically]

Even though it was a bit sore and it was – maybe more difficult for the student, you were happy to – just – ah – let them – practice on you.

'Specially when the needle's up there and they're doing this with it. [He mimes the student wiggling the needle from side to side to get it into the vein.]

An empathic response

During our interview, Peter's demeanour suggests that he is enjoying our dialogue, and I laugh at his dry wit several times. When I read the transcript of this first patient interview, I noticed that I interrupted him several times and could have listened more carefully. In this excerpt, I repeatedly ask what it was like for him being interviewed or examined by students and he insists that he didn't mind, even if their examination caused some discomfort. From his stories, it seems that our interview serves a different purpose for him than it does for me. Rather than describing his own experience of each interaction, he focuses on his appraisal of the students, and as a result he constructs his identity in relation to them.

In his vivid description of a particular time students approached him, he says they were 'standing around on one leg'. He represents them as child-like, by adopting a whining tone of voice, and associating their behaviour with that of his children. When he says that 'a few of them were game to poke and prod' (meaning to examine his abdomen), his choice of words is telling. By using the word 'game' he implies that they had to muster a degree of courage, while the phrase 'poke and prod' suggests that their efforts were unskilled or clumsy. Despite this, he claims he was not concerned because 'they couldn't really hurt me that bad'.

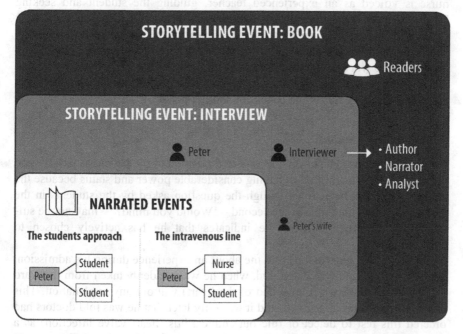

Figure 4.1 Peter's story: multi-level analysis.

In relation to the timid, inept and naïve identity he constructs for the students, he identifies himself as confident, stoic and agreeable, like an indulgent father. As I mentioned earlier, stories are often animated by fears and desires of the narrator or other story characters (Frank, 2010; Lemke, 2008). In this story, Peter is in a position of power in relation to the students, because they need his agreement to examine him – something which students can both desire and fear. He is willing to help and unconcerned by the potential to increase his own discomfort, because, as he puts it, 'they've gotta learn, haven't they?' Peter's response could be characterised as one of empathy, because he imagines the emotions of the students and acts to alleviate their unease.

In the second passage, Peter describes a time when a student inserted an intravenous line into his arm with the help of a nurse. Although this caused significant pain, he insists that he was pleased to help. He told this story in response to a question about how students introduce themselves. I was interested in how open they were with patients about their status as students. For Peter this was not really an issue; all that mattered was that the student 'was there for training'. After she fails at her initial attempt, he can tell that she is 'very embarrassed'.

At this point I ask how he had felt about having a student do the procedure. He does not reply, and it is unclear whether he fails to hear my interruption or decides to ignore it. He continues with his story, describing how the student asked for the nurse's help after her initial attempt. An exchange is reported between Peter and the nurse, but he does not report the student's speech. The nurse is voiced as an experienced teacher, guiding the student and seeking Peter's consent on her behalf for a further attempt. Peter identifies himself in relation to the nurse as her associate in support of the student, who eventually succeeded with his help and that of the nurse. His ironic tone in response to my question as to whether the procedure hurt him may be his way of conveying that it was quite painful. He identifies himself as stoic, by describing how he tolerated considerable pain for the benefit of another person.

Shifting power relations

Peter's stories reveal a shift in the expected position of the patient as passive and vulnerable. He is identified as having considerable power and status because the students need his help. Even though the question asked by the students in the first passage and the nurse in the second – 'Would you mind?' – may not be sufficient for informed consent, he indicates that he has actively chosen to participate.

Earlier in the interview he told me about an experience during his admission, before his condition was diagnosed, when he was suddenly taken from the ward for an echocardiogram (ultrasound of the heart) without any explanation. This made him feel very concerned, and it was only later that he was told doctors had ordered this test to detect or rule out endocarditis (heart valve infection) as a cause for his mysterious fever. When this story is juxtaposed with those about his encounters with students, it suggests another potential reason for his willingness to help them. In addition to a genuine desire to help, he is also likely to have gained a sense of agency, which is integral to his identity construction within the interview. This interpretation emerges only when the analysis extends to include the context in which the narrative is told (Wortham, 2001).

Resisting identity disruption

The next story is from my interview with a patient named Harvey and tells about a different kind of experience with students. Like Peter, Harvey identifies himself in relation to the students – and his interviewer – through storytelling in a research interview. Like all stories, Harvey's were designed for a particular audience – in this case, me as his interviewer. Like all participants in this study, Harvey knew I was a doctor as well as a researcher. At the time of the interview, he was recovering from an acute episode of heart failure, which was the reason for this admission to hospital. I had met him earlier at a bedside tutorial, during which he seemed to enjoy telling the group quite a few long and convoluted stories.

During the interview, I sat beside his bed, while he reclined on top of it. Just like most shared rooms in acute hospitals, it was a rather chaotic environment. Although I was the primary audience for his stories and his partner in conversation, there were others in the room either continuously or intermittently, including nurses and other patients, most of whom were attached to intravenous pumps. Any of these people and non-human *agents* (such as the IV pumps) might have influenced Harvey's story production and performance. Nurses came in and out of the room every few minutes to check on other patients or respond to the incessant beeping of their intravenous pumps, all the while engaging loudly in conversation with patients or each other.

At one point, a team of doctors arrived on their ward round, and I stepped out of the room while they reviewed his medical status. From time to time, emergency announcements were heard over the public-address system. Sometimes, the noise and activity provoked pauses or repetitions in our dialogue, and we had to work hard to stay focused. At the start of the interview, one of the beds and its occupant were missing. Later, a visitor came in and asked if anyone knew where that patient might be, and Harvey told her he had gone for an X-ray. He appeared to feel at home in this place, with the confident air of an experienced patient.

Early in the interview, Harvey began to tell me about an episode that took place years before, when he was diagnosed with Legionnaire's disease, a serious respiratory infection. He associated that illness with his current heart condition, and the story spoke of his resilience and previous experience of hospitalisation. However, it was never finished because I interrupted him just as he was about to tell me about his admission to the intensive care unit, changing the topic to inquire about his interactions with students.

Just before telling me the story that follows, Harvey told me he was amused by the hesitant manner of students listening to his heart. He said that, having been examined so often by doctors, he knew exactly where the students needed to place their stethoscopes. I asked whether he had ever felt uncomfortable with students and he produced the story below about a student he perceived as arrogant. Subsequently, he told me how an 'arrogant doctor' made an error of judgement in his treatment of Harvey after he suffered an injury as a teenager, and how Harvey had been right to contradict him. Although he showed no outward sign that he was offended by my disrespectful interruption of his Legionnaire's disease story, I believe it is relevant to the analysis of the material that followed. It also highlights parallels between student-patient encounters and the interaction between myself as researcher and Harvey as participant, especially the ways in which identities can be contested.

Doing that 'one-upmanship'

Do you ever get uncomfortable [interacting with students]?

Oh yeah, I had one bloke – one bloke that I was uncomfortable with.

Mm – what happened?

Because – I sort of got the feeling that the only reason he listened to me chest was because a couple of others had. And he thought: 'Well, I'll show them what I can do', type of thing, with it. And that was the way he acted towards me when he put the stethoscope on. It wasn't: 'I'm putting the stethoscope here because this is where I want to hear from'. It was 'This looks about the right place', type of thing.

Just like a bit of a routine?

Yeah, type of thing, yeah. Just – yeah.

You were just uncomfortable?

Yeah, it just wasn't – you know, it didn't feel as if I was helping him; it was as if he was trying to take –

[Loud conversation between nurses in the background. He pauses in mid-sentence]

– not so much from me, but get a – a boost on all the other ones that were there.

It didn't feel like he was accepting your help, like, that you were offering.

No – he just – to me, he just felt like – he thought he was the boss of all those students.

He thought he was better than the others?

Yeah, and so: 'I'll do this, but I'll show them that I'm better at it', and that. And in the end, in the end he got a bit of a shock because – he asked me a question and I just said to him, 'No'. And he looked at me –

What was the question?

Oh, I can't think. It was something – um – 'Was I right?' or something, and that. You know, as much as to – he was expecting me to say – 'Oh yeah, you did that perfectly' or something, type of thing. And I just went: 'No'.

He would've got a bit of a surprise.

I turned to the girl and said, 'Would you like it – would you like to listen?' And that.

Yeah, OK. So, you were pretty displeased with his approach.

I was displeased with his approach, and – soon as he opened his mouth enough that I could – cut 'im [emphatically] – I did.

Yeah, OK. [Interviewer laughs]

I mean, I don't know if that was the right thing to do or the wrong thing to do.

It just felt right to you at the time.

Yeah, I just didn't want him trying to be a one up – do a one-upmanship, and using me to do that one-upmanship. Yeah – on the rest of his class.

So, was he kind of using you?

That's what I felt – that he was trying to use me to get one up on all his classmates, type of thing.

And you didn't like that.

No, I don't like people like that.

But most of the students, if they're really listening to you – you don't get the feeling like they're using you?

No. They haven't – he's the only one I ever felt – got the feeling that I was being used by. I've got some that I've just thought: 'Nah, they're not going to make it. No, they're not the right person to be a doctor', type of thing, and that. But I won't try and shoot them down. Because to me, that's not up to me. That's up to the doc – their teachers, themselves or – they might talk to someone and [snaps his fingers] click into it and do it right.

Yeah – they've got a chance to improve.

Yeah. Where – this bloke was just trying to – I mean, I don't doubt that he wanted to be a doctor; but – he thought he was going to be the doctor.

Yeah, I get what you mean, yeah. [Interviewer laughs]

I don't – I'm not – I'm not here to try and – boost someone's ego, [Harvey laughs] I'm afraid, you know.

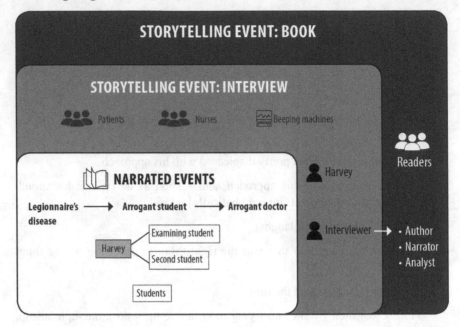

Figure 4.2 Harvey's story: multi-level analysis.

A moral judgement

This excerpt tells about an extraordinary event – the only time Harvey has ever felt uncomfortable during his interactions with medical students. Harvey identifies himself as a shrewd judge of character, who acts decisively to avoid one student in a group taking advantage of his generosity at the expense of the others. A negative moral judgement of the student's character is implied when he insists that he would not respond in the same way to students who merely seem to lack aptitude. Describing his response to the student's behaviour, he identifies himself as assertive and aware of his power to withdraw co-operation from the students at any time. It was only later that I realised this could apply just as well to his participation in our interview.

Harvey's manner of speech, with a broad Australian accent and redundant phrases at the end of many sentences ('type of thing'; 'and that'), identify his origins as working-class. He implies that he has had limited educational opportunities compared with medical students and his interviewer. At one stage, he says: 'I'm not Mr Knowledgeable, but I think if I'm willing to talk to you, you should be willing to listen to me'. He is adamant that his lack of education does not reduce his entitlement to respect.

Harvey's narrative performance conveys how he perceives himself in relation to the medical profession and its students, especially in terms of social status. Rather than referring explicitly to status or social class, Harvey alludes to them through his colourful use of metaphorical expressions. He expresses the difference in social status between individuals or groups in terms of relative height or elevation, revealing an underlying conceptual metaphor (Kövecses, 2010). This was also observed in a previous study of the metaphors used to characterise doctor-patient relationships (Rees, Knight, & Wilkinson, 2007).

To express his judgement that the student examining him was trying to make himself out to be better than the others, Harvey said he was 'trying to do a one-upmanship', 'get a boost on the others there', and 'get one up on his classmates'. He says in relation to the offending student that he 'cut 'im' – arguably meaning cut him down to size; and that he is not there to 'boost someone's ego'. He insists that he would not 'shoot down' students who seem unsuitable for other reasons.

The offending student is voiced as an arrogant, selfish person. Harvey reports what he believes the student is thinking in the form of direct speech: 'Well, I'll show them what I can do' and 'I'll do this, but I'll show them I'm better at it'. This represents another instance of ventriloquation: speaking through another person's words or, in this case, their imagined thoughts. Harvey employs this technique to construct the student's identity as arrogant (Wortham, 2001). He goes on to say that the student was 'expecting' him to say that he had done the examination perfectly, and 'using me to do that one-upmanship'. These remarks serve a rhetorical function, characterising the student as manipulative, so that Harvey's response is more likely to be seen as justified.

As he tells the story, Harvey voices himself as an active agent in his interaction with the students, pursuing his own agenda. He emphasises his aversion to being exploited or treated as if he were inferior. Class differences may have influenced his reaction to the student; prior research has shown they can affect how doctors and patients relate to each other (Roter & Hall, 2006).

Disrupting identity work

Speaking about his reaction to the student, Harvey says: 'I don't know if that was the right thing to do or the wrong thing to do', suggesting a degree of ambivalence. In addition to social class differences, the identity work of the student-patient interaction may also have contributed to the exchange. The way Harvey explains his discomfort implies that his efforts to construct and perform his preferred identity were disrupted by the student's behaviour. He says that: 'it didn't feel as if I was helping him; it was as if he was trying to take ... not so much from me, but get a boost on all the other ones that were there'. The identity Harvey wants to construct and perform in relation to the students is that of an experienced patient, generously offering to help their learning. Perceiving that the student is taking from the others rather than accepting Harvey's generosity may be interpreted as a denial of his preferred identity.

To enable Harvey to construct and perform that identity, the students must identify themselves as worthy recipients of his help. The denial of his preferred identity may have contributed to his feeling of being used or exploited. He makes it clear that trying to advance one's own position in relation to the rest of the group is not consistent with his purpose; he is not there 'to boost someone's ego'. He withdraws his co-operation from the first student and offers it to another, asking: 'Would you like to listen?' In doing so, he performs the identity as a generous helper that the first student's behaviour appeared to threaten.

Harvey's narrative treatment of the student provides an opportunity for reflection on what it means to relate to another person in a dialogic way. Bakhtin's 'moral ideal of human relations as dialogue' (Frank, 2004, p. 43) was originally described in relation to character development by authors of fiction. He later demonstrated that it is relevant to all human interactions. From a narrative perspective, a dialogic story is one in which the voice of one or more characters can be recognised as distinct from that of the author. The narrator tells the story using the voice of the character or characters, rather than only using their own voice to tell the reader about them. Extending this idea to everyday life, if I am to relate to others dialogically, I must consider their perspectives as well as my own, including their interpretation of my own actions (Frank, 2004).

During the interview, Harvey acts as the narrator, but also a character in the stories he tells. He does not reflect on how other characters in the story might interpret his actions, and nor does he consider alternative interpretations of the actions of the student who offends him. In Bakhtinian terms, he seeks to *finalise* that student: that is, to define what he is and limit what he can become (Frank, 2004). In this respect, he treats him differently from other characters in the story – including other students he has judged to be unsuitable. In their case, he leaves open the possibility that they will prove him wrong; in other words, they are *unfinalised*.

Like Broyard writing about his doctor, and Peter earlier in this chapter, Harvey inverts the usual power relations between patients and health professionals (Broyard, 1992). However, he does so at the expense of the student, because he makes a negative judgement about his character. Harvey's story reminds us of the inherently moral quality of storytelling, because his objection to the offending student's behaviour and his defence of his own response are framed in terms of moral norms (Nelson, 2001).

By taking a stance in relation to the actions or speech of another character in a story, narrators 'express evaluations of social experience' and 'convey their position on a variety of social problems ... without openly asserting their views' (De Fina, Schiffrin, & Bamberg, 2006, p. 11). Both Peter and Harvey's stories can be said to take such a position in relation to the characters with whom they interact.

It is feasible that Harvey believed the student came from a privileged background, predisposing him to perceive him as arrogant. This perception might also apply to his assessment of me in the research interview. During the interview, Harvey displays ambivalence towards doctors in several stories: some of his remarks indicate respect while others reveal his belief that doctors tend to be self-important. His story about an encounter with an 'arrogant' doctor 50 years earlier offers some insight into why he may have told the 'arrogant student' story during our interview.

Identity construction in the research interview

In many respects, a research interview is analogous to a clinical teaching encounter. The overt reason for patients to interact with medical students is that they are in a unique position to share their stories and offer their bodies for examination. However, clinical teaching encounters take on a variety of other meanings for patients who participate in them (Chretien et al., 2010; McLachlan, King, Wenger, & Dornan, 2012; Rice, 2008). This means they may have a range of possible reasons for deciding whether to see students or not, on a particular occasion. Some patients have described these interactions as events to be tolerated, expecting no personal benefit; others experience satisfaction from helping, or perceive them as opportunities to learn about their condition. Being in hospital can be tedious, involving a lot of waiting around with nothing to do, and an interaction with students can make some patients feel that people are interested in and care about them. These interpretations can change over the course of an interaction, depending, at least in part, on the extent to which the patient is engaged in dialogue (Chretien et al., 2010).

Similarly, the supposed reason for research participants to agree to an interview is to contribute to the project and help the researcher. However, like patients' encounters with medical students, research interviews are also sites for social interaction and identity construction (Tanggaard, 2009; Wortham, 2000).

When Harvey tells me his story about the student who made him feel uncomfortable, he also constructs and performs his identity in relation to me, his interviewer. Early in the interview he says: 'I think, if I'm willing to talk to you, you should be willing to listen to me'. This statement is made in the context of a discussion about how some students seem not to pay attention when he speaks to them. However, I reflect later that it takes on another meaning in relation to his interaction with me. He is saying that, in return for his storytelling he expects to receive genuine attention from his audience. This is especially significant because I had previously cut short his story about Legionnaire's disease, an intervention which I believe may have influenced the rest of the interview.

After telling me the story about the student who made him feel uncomfortable, Harvey said that he found students in general to be more attentive than doctors, and then remarked: 'You'll always get your arrogant doctors'. Then he began a long and detailed account of an encounter in his youth with a doctor who Harvey thought behaved towards him in an arrogant way. His purpose in telling me that story was not immediately obvious. At first, it appeared to be to support his assertion that the first doctor in the story had been arrogant on the grounds that Harvey had been correct – according to a specialist he saw later – when he had disagreed with the first doctor's diagnosis. But telling the story also accomplished substantial identity work.

Through it, he identified himself as a former police cadet from a small country town, who already had some of the ambivalence towards doctors and medical authority that he demonstrated in the present day. He told me how, even at the age of 16, he had challenged a locum doctor whose opinion he disagreed with but that he had also been impressed by a 'top specialist'. I do not know whether he went on to become a police officer; but if this were the case, he would have been accustomed to considerable power and authority. It might also have contributed to his strong sense of agency, and his reaction to the perception that he was being used for a morally suspect purpose.

Although it is not possible to be certain about the relationship between the three stories told by Harvey and depicted in Figure 4.2, I believe there may have been a link between them. It was after I terminated Harvey's story about his Legionnaire's disease episode that he told me about his encounter with the 'arrogant' student. Soon after this, he brought up the tale of the arrogant doctor. After listening to my recording of the interview and noticing with regret my disrespectful interruption, I realised that all of these stories contributed to Harvey's identity construction. It is feasible that the impulse to construct and perform his identity was one factor motivating him to agree to be interviewed. My interruption of the first story temporarily restricted his performance, but he had many other tales to tell during the interview. This can be understood as another instance of *emergence*, showing yet again how, when we are focusing on the analysis of a particular story, we need to take the context in which it is told into account because this often provides further insight into the meanings of the story under consideration.

Relating dialogically

A research interview is not simply an occasion for telling stories that already exist in the mind of the participant; instead, it is a 'setting for the dialogical production of personal narratives and social life' (Tanggaard, 2009, p. 1499). From this explicitly Bakhtinian perspective, meanings are 'performed in a borderline area between oneself and others' (Tanggaard, 2009, p. 1500). Bakhtin's view was that human beings construct themselves by attempting to see, through another's eyes, aspects of themselves that they are otherwise unable to perceive (Frank, 2004). Each person has a *surplus of seeing* in relationship to the other. We need to maintain our awareness of the difference between our own and another's view of the world, if we are to relate dialogically to that person.

If we fail to recognise this, there is a risk we will come to perceive a reality defined by our own needs and priorities, and 'we feel ourselves justified in acting on this reality' (Frank, 2004, p. 45). Harvey's response to the offending student is an example of a *monologic* way of relating. He expresses certainty as to the intentions and character of the student in question, and the doctor in his later story, therefore *finalising* them (Frank, 2004). In view of his assessment of the student, he feels justified in taking retribution by withdrawing his co-operation, in a way that may have puzzled and embarrassed the student.

When I brought Harvey's 'Legionnaire's disease' story to a premature close to pursue my own agenda, my intervention was like that of a student who cuts off a patient's story when they seem to be straying from the intended path of the interview. I gave insufficient attention to the meanings conveyed by that story because I was thinking about the data I wished to collect, just as medical students often focus too narrowly on the path to a diagnosis. Decades of medical practice may have predisposed me to interrupt others in the pursuit of what I consider to be vital data; this is a pitfall for students and clinicians as well as researchers. This was a salient lesson for me about listening to participants and being respectful of their agenda, as well as my own. It was also a reminder of what it means to relate dialogically, and to reflect on how the other person might be interpreting my interaction with them.

Reflecting later about how I had interacted with Harvey, I wonder how he might have described our interview to another person (Frank, 2004). Would he have characterised my disruption of his story about his Legionnaire's disease merely as inattentive; or worse, the conduct of another arrogant doctor? His continuing co-operation with me for the rest of the interview suggests he was not too deeply offended. However, I wonder whether his long-winded story of the 'arrogant doctor' may have been a test of my willingness to pay attention. Despite my uncertainty at the time as to why he was telling it, I stayed and listened attentively until the end, and I hope that was sufficient to redeem myself in his eyes.

Both Peter and Harvey construct identities relationally, through their assessment of students' character, emotions or motivations and their own position in relation to them. My findings build on previous research showing that for some patients, their encounters with students have social and relational implications (Chretien et al., 2010). Thinking about identity work, power dynamics and social status can reveal deeper meanings of a story told in a given context. Patients are often willing to help students learn, but they may expect something in return. To meet their expectations requires some insight into what they might hope for, and a willingness to explore and address each patient's agenda alongside that of the student or teacher. Awareness of the self-identifying function of stories should contribute to a better appreciation of their importance.

Regrettably, some patients involved in students' learning can feel as though they have been treated like an inanimate object. At other times they can feel like an active participant or offer ideas as to how this might be accomplished. In the next chapter, I explore this tension through patients' stories about how they felt they were treated in clinical teaching encounters.

References

Bleakley, A., & Bligh, J. (2008). Students learning from patients: Let's get real in medical education. *Advances in Health Sciences Education, 13*, 89–107.

Broyard, A. (1992). *Intoxicated by my illness and other writings on life and mortality.* New York: Clarkson Potter.

Chretien, K., Goldman, E., Craven, K., & Faselis, C. (2010). A qualitative study of the meaning of physical examination teaching for patients. *Journal of General Internal Medicine, 25*(8), 786–791.

De Fina, A., Schiffrin, D., & Bamberg, M. (Eds.). (2006). *Discourse and identity*. Cambridge: Cambridge University Press.

Fletcher, K., Furney, S., & Stern, D. (2007). Patients speak: What's really important about bedside interactions with physician teams. *Teaching and Learning in Medicine, 19*(2), 120–127.

Fletcher, K., Rankey, D., & Stern, D. (2005). Bedside interactions from the other side of the bedrail. *Journal of General Internal Medicine, 20*, 58–61.

Frank, A. W. (2002). 'How can they act like that?' Physicians and patients as characters in each other's stories. *Hastings Center Report, 32*(6), 14–22.

Frank, A. W. (2004). *The renewal of generosity: Illness, medicine and how to live*. Chicago, IL: The University of Chicago Press.

Frank, A. W. (2010). *Letting stories breathe: A socio-narratology*. Chicago, IL & London: University of Chicago Press.

Goldie, J. (2012). The formation of professional identity in medical students: Considerations for educators. *Medical Teacher, 34*, e641–e648.

Kövecses, Z. (2010). *Metaphor: A practical introduction* (2nd ed.). New York: Oxford University Press.

Lemke, J. L. (2008). Identity, development and desire: Critical questions. In C. R. Caldas-Coulthard & R. Iedema (Eds.), *Identity trouble: Critical discourse and contested identities* (pp. 17–42). Basingstoke & New York: Palgrave Macmillan.

McLachlan, E., King, N., Wenger, E., & Dornan, T. (2012). Phenomenological analysis of patient experiences of medical student teaching encounters. *Medical Education, 46*(10), 963–973. doi:10.1111/j.1365-2923.2012.04332.x

Murchison, J. M. (2010). *Ethnography essentials*. San Francisco, CA: Jossey-Bass.

Nair, B. R., Coughlan, J. L., & Hensley, M. J. (1997). Student and patient perspectives on bedside teaching. *Medical Education, 31*, 341–346.

Nelson, H. L. (2001). *Damaged identities: Narrative repair*. Ithaca, NY & London: Cornell University Press.

Rees, C., Knight, L., & Wilkinson, C. (2007). Doctors being up there and we being down there: A metaphorical analysis of talk about student/doctor relationships. *Social Science and Medicine, 65*, 725–737.

Rice, T. (2008). 'Beautiful murmurs': Stethoscopic listening and acoustic objectification. *The Senses and Society, 3*, 293–306. doi:10.2752/174589308X331332

Romano, J. (1941). Patients' attitudes and behavior in ward round teaching. *JAMA (Chicago, Ill.), 117*(9), 664–667.

Roter, D., & Hall, J. (2006). *Doctors talking with patients/patients talking with doctors: Improving communication in medical visits* (2nd ed.). Westport, CT: Praeger.

Salmon, P., & Young, B. (2011). Creativity in clinical communication: From communication skills to skilled communication. *Medical Education, 45*, 217–226.

Tanggaard, L. (2009). The research interview as a dialogical context for the production of social life and personal narratives. *Qualitative Inquiry, 15*(9), 1498–1515.

Wortham, S. (2000). Interactional positioning and narrative self-construction. *Narrative Inquiry, 10*(1), 157–184. doi:10.1075/ni.10.1.11wor

Wortham, S. (2001). *Narratives in action: A strategy for research and analysis*. New York: Teachers College Press.

Wortham, S. (2006). *Learning identity: The joint emergence of social identification and academic learning*. New York: Cambridge University Press.

5   Object or active participant?

Did you have the feeling that you were being thought of as a person?
That is a good question. I think with their attitude I am happy. Whether they see
me as an object of learning or as a human person, I think I'm happy with that. As
long as their attitude's nice, kind and sensitive I'm OK with it. The personal
element of – really understand me as a person, I think is not that strongly present
in that environment. I may be wrong, but it depends on how students see themselves when they come to see a patient. But from my point of view, they just
want to get something out of it and that's it.

Yuan, patient in medical ward

Patient participation in clinical teaching

Yuan says he is happy to help students by participating in their learning, as
long as they treat him kindly. However, he feels that they are only focused on
what they can get from the interaction, and not on understanding him as a
person. He observes that the way students treat him depends on *how they see
themselves*, showing great insight and highlighting the relational dimension of
identities.

This chapter is based on patient stories about teaching and learning encounters, including some in which they felt treated like an inanimate object. There
has been some published research exploring patients' perspectives on their participation in students' learning (McLachlan, King, Wenger, & Dornan, 2012;
Monrouxe, Rees, & Bradley, 2009; Towle et al., 2010). The stories in this
chapter reveal that some common ways of involving patients in clinical teaching
tend to promote feelings of objectification while others are more likely to foster
a sense of collaboration. This knowledge should inform the development of
teaching practices that respect patients' needs, alongside those of students
(Chretien, Goldman, Craven, & Faselis, 2010).

Robin's story offers insight into some of the ways in which patients experience their participation in clinical teaching. Robin was a middle-aged immigrant
from the United Kingdom whom I met during a bedside tutorial. He had been
admitted a few days earlier with life-threatening bleeding from the stomach,
causing him to vomit blood. Before the students entered, the tutor asked Robin if

he would let one of them ask him some questions, and she told him exactly what she would like him to do. The student would ask him questions about his illness, but they would only be allowed eight minutes, and she wanted him to respond without volunteering any additional information. As I listened to his interaction with the student, it emerged that after a similar haemorrhage some years earlier, he had been advised never to take aspirin again, because it could precipitate another episode. However, a few months before this admission, he had been prescribed aspirin for a heart condition and had believed it was only a matter of time before it caused another haemorrhage.

Robin agreed to being interviewed the next day for my research, but we were interrupted by the arrival of his lunch. When I returned, he told me his doctor had visited him on the ward round, and two students had been to see him as well. He explained that this ward round had been different from the others. Previously, the doctors stood around at the end of his bed, speaking to each other using technical terms that he could not understand. He had felt unable to ask questions, because they came and went too quickly. But this time, and in his opinion partly because of the chair I had placed beside his bed, the doctor had decided to sit down, and Robin had his concerns addressed for the first time. That part of his story is presented and discussed in Chapter 2.

The following exchange was prompted by a question about how his interactions with students in a tutorial with a clinical teacher compared with the times students came on their own.

Well, there's no real difference. I mean, I must say the one where the doctor was with them … and one had to – she came and asked me – that, I think, was the one where I saw you – and then she said 'Don't lead them in'. … Yeah, that was quite interesting.

So, because you knew what was expected and you were supposed to hold back a bit of information, did you feel more, a bit like a teacher or something in that setting?

Well I felt more part of it rather than just being the object of, you know, 'Oh let's just use him because he's here'.

So, does it sometimes feel a little bit like that?

Oh, it does. [Emphatically]

You're a bit of an object to be used?

Well yeah, yeah. They're saying: 'You're a captive audience' and if you won't say 'Yes, I don't mind'. That's it. 'OK, let's go'.

But what made it feel less like that was involving you more?

Yeah. Like, 'Only answer the questions. Don't forward information that they're not going to be asking'.

And what was it like when the students examined you? Did they look after your comfort and stuff like that?

Well, they were a bit clumsy.

So, did they hurt you at all or –?

Well <u>yeah</u>, because um – I think they don't <u>know</u> that – I mean <u>I'm</u> OK because I haven't <u>got</u> any pain. But like, you know, they would <u>press.</u>

Push a bit too hard – harder than you'd expect?

Yeah. It's like, because they haven't done it before. That type of thing, you know.

Alright and … have you got the impression that they were interested in what the experience of being sick was like for <u>you,</u> how you felt about it? Does that ever come up when they're talking to you?

No. I must say that it's almost – and <u>I don't mind,</u> but – you're the piece of equipment that they're just using to get what they have to get. Yeah?

In this excerpt, Robin explains that the tutor describing what she wanted him to do made him feel like a participant, whereas on other occasions he felt more like an object. He was not too concerned about students' examinations being clumsy even though they did hurt, saying: 'I'm OK, because I haven't got any

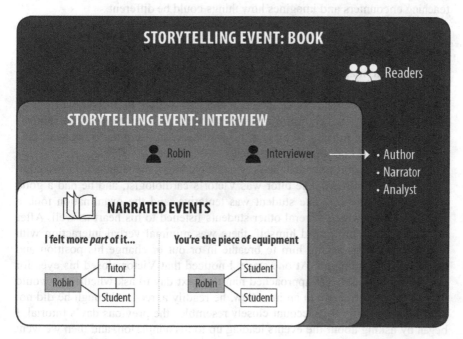

Figure 5.1 Robin's story: multi-level analysis.

pain'. He does not think students are interested in his experience of illness, but that they see him as a 'piece of equipment they're just using to get what they have to get'. Robin identifies himself as an altruistic and stoic man, because he is willing to help despite the clumsy examinations and being treated as an object. He uses direct speech to represent the tutor's advice to him: 'Don't forward information that they're not going to be asking'. By speaking through the tutor's words, he employs the narrative device of ventriloquation. In doing so, he identifies her as a respectful professional, and he responds by feeling like 'part of it'.

He also uses direct speech and ventriloquation to represent the students' thoughts, as he imagines them: 'Let's just use him because he's here'. He identifies them as self-centred and inconsiderate, implying he has little choice about whether to see them because he is 'a captive audience'. Robin's demeanour is cheerful, despite telling me that he has felt objectified in some of his interactions with students, and that they are not interested in his experience. Although he is willing to go along with being used for their benefit, he critically evaluates students' character and competence, depicting them as inconsiderate and clumsy.

Previous research into patient involvement in clinical education has emphasised the benefits of clinical teachers explaining to patients what would be expected of them before the event (Chretien et al., 2010; Fletcher, Furney, & Stern, 2007; Nair, Coughlan, & Hensley, 1997; Romano, 1941). Robin's positive response to the tutor's approach lends support to this recommendation, but his remark that it was unusual resonates with my own observations in the field.

In the next story, another patient describes how he has felt during clinical teaching encounters and imagines how things could be different.

Looking for courage and connection

Victor was a married man with teenage children, originally from Eastern Europe, so English was not his first language. He had been admitted for investigation of a possible heart valve infection and was waiting to find out whether he would need surgery. The murmur associated with his condition, mitral stenosis (narrowing of the mitral valve), is difficult to hear, so listening to his heart presented a valuable opportunity for students.

During a tutorial I attended the previous day, one of the students was asked to listen to Victor's heart. The tutor was Victor's cardiologist, and he had a good relationship with him. The student was tentative, and the examination took a long time, after which several other students listened to his heart as well. After the student had introduced himself, there was minimal verbal interaction with Victor, apart from asking him to breathe in or out or change his position and thanking him at the end. At one stage, I noticed that Victor closed his eyes for several minutes. When I approached him the next day to ask whether he would be willing to participate in an interview, he readily agreed. Although he did not refer to it explicitly, his account closely resembles the previous day's tutorial. I began by asking about the events leading up to his admission, and then we went on to talk about his experiences with students.

So, I'm interested in knowing what it feels like for you to have the students coming to see you.

Oh – um – oh – I was – um – happy. I'm not worried. Um – if they ask me if they want to listen, or they want to check up, I'm happy to let them – do it because that's how they learn. If – if – if – if I say no, how would they know how to – what to look for if somebody else is sick, and they are GPs, they are going to be GPs or whatever they are going to be, and then they check somebody and they are not sure, or they haven't heard that one before? How can they compare, how can they make the diagnostic right if they – if you learn in school or in uni and they say, 'Oh, this is what you should hear' or whatever, but if they didn't really hear it in real life? How would they know what to listen to? So, I'm happy, if they come, they want to listen – it's all right.

And, while they're actually listening to you, does it feel like – they're thinking about you as a person, or does it feel like they're just concentrating on your heart or the sounds that they're hearing – do you think about that?

[Long pause] Probably. The thing is that they are – I think a bit – how you call it – they are not really comfortable – probably, maybe they are a bit – not scared, but –

Yeah, they're a bit nervous?

Yeah, they are. And they don't – they don't – I think, they don't have much courage. To tell – to tell the patient what to do or – like, I can –

So, you don't know what they want from you?

Yeah, not exactly because they're not very clear in what they want. They don't say it. [Taps hand on table for emphasis] I'm not sure if in class they practise – I've read that they practise one on one, like student to student, but that's a different thing; because I can choose someone like a friend, and I'm very comfortable with them, with him or her and then, I can tell her or him what to do. And you can be clear and comfortable to tell them what to do. But when they come here, they don't know me, and then they try – they don't have the courage to tell me what to do and I need to – I want them to tell me what to do. [Emphatic] Like, if they want me to sit up, tell me to sit up. If they want me to breathe, tell me to breathe, and tell me to stop breathing but then tell me to start breathing again.

Start breathing again! [Interviewer laughs] So you don't go blue?

Yeah, because I'm waiting! [Victor laughs] 'Cause they say, 'Stop breathing'. I'll stop, but then they have to tell me that – 'Breathe normally'. [Both laugh]

So, you notice from them that the instructions are not very clear.

Not yet. They don't have enough courage – and enough confidence to – they are not so sure about themselves. Because – and a little bit – not stressed out, but nervous. 'Am I doing the right thing or – because too many people here, watching, what am I doing'. Yeah, so a bit hard for the one guy doing it. Yeah, and that's the one thing, which one, yeah. That they – they should be more confident. I know it's hard when you see a person and you've never met them before, but if you are going to be a doctor you have to be – just – just – have the courage to talk to them straight and loud enough for them to hear you, what you want from them. [Interviewer laughs]

Do you think the students that you saw, do you think they were always thinking … are they thinking about you, are they thinking about if you're comfortable? Or more are they thinking about how nervous they feel?

Mm – I don't think they really think about me like a patient, they think about me like a – like a something you use to learn on. It's not really like a person; doesn't look like they feel, or they have that human feeling for you. It's like, oh – I'm just like a dummy. Not really a dummy dummy, but like a human dummy, which one you can experiment on.

So – is there something that you would perhaps like them to do differently? So that you felt they relate more like a person, to you? What would make it different?

If they – before, let's say – get to know the person a little bit. Not really all your whatever, whatever, you know, just couple questions or something, just to get a little bit to know the person. I think, like make them feel that you are – they are interested in you like a person. Not just 'Oh – this is the test dummy. We just use them to listen and learn something from it and that's it'. So, I think that a bit more connecting – connecting with the patient.

And so, do you think … they have any idea about what you're going through; about your experience?

[Long pause] Probably, but not the full extent. Probably they understand the medical condition, what you are going through. But there is all other stuff behind it, there is emotional and other stuff, which one, I don't think they get to that level. They are just 'Oh, this is the diagnostic and that's really it'.

Victor's story is represented below in three parts, which are discussed in the text along with the results of the analysis.

In the first part, I ask Victor what it feels like when students come to see him. He hesitates and uses filler words in his answer: 'Oh – um – oh – I was – um – happy'. This suggests a degree of ambivalence, which may be better understood in the light of his later revelations. He goes on to explain: 'If I say no, how would they know … what to look for if somebody else is sick …?' Victor implies he feels a sense of obligation, not only to the students but to their future patients. He acknowledges that the only way to learn how to recognise a heart murmur is to hear it 'in real life'. He decides that the benefits to others justify his own potential discomfort, identifying himself as an altruistic person.

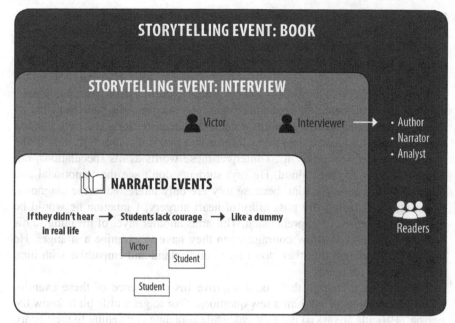

STORYTELLING EVENT: BOOK

STORYTELLING EVENT: INTERVIEW

Victor   Interviewer ⟶ • Author
• Narrator
• Analyst

Readers

NARRATED EVENTS

If they didn't hear ⟶ Students lack courage ⟶ Like a dummy
in real life

Victor
Student
Student

Figure 5.2 Victor's story: multi-level analysis.

In the second part, he does not answer directly when I ask if he thinks students see him as a person but says they 'don't have enough courage – and enough confidence' to explain what they want from him. He describes how a student asked him to stop breathing so he could hear the murmur more clearly, but did not tell him when he could breathe again. He tells the story with an amused tone of voice but implies that it was unpleasant at the time.

Victor recognises it is harder for students to examine him than to practise on their peers, and difficult to perform a challenging task with people watching. Like Peter in Chapter 4, he portrays students as timid and apprehensive. He also evaluates them critically, saying: 'if you are going to be a doctor you have to … have the courage to talk to them straight and loud enough for them to hear you'. In this part of the story, Victor speaks with the voice of a responsible adult, like a father or teacher, expressing both empathy and constructive criticism. I reflect that Victor's children may be only a few years younger than these students; this might help him imagine how they might be feeling.

In the third part of the story, I ask again whether Victor thinks students are interested in how he is feeling. He answers this time, using the word *dummy* to express how he felt during the examination. The word can refer to a mannequin or ventriloquist's doll but also has connotations of low intelligence or an inability to speak. He initially says 'I'm just like a dummy' then goes on to say that a dummy is 'one you can experiment on' and that he does not want to be seen as 'the test dummy'. This suggests that the examination makes him feel like a passive subject of experimentation. As I reflect later that he made this remark during our research interview, I hope our conversation did not make him feel this way as well. The term dummy can also refer to a replica or imitation, so it has links with the idea of the simulacrum, as discussed in Chapter 3. Victor might be feeling that he was treated as a likeness of a person, rather than the real thing.

Victor's depiction of students echoes Robin's portrayal of them as uninterested in his well-being or emotional state. He too presents their thoughts as direct speech, using ventriloquation to construct identities for them: 'We just use them to listen and learn something from it and that's it', and: 'Oh, this is the diagnostic and that's really it'. I interpret these words as his speculations, not that anyone spoke them aloud. He says students don't see the 'emotional and other stuff' going on for him, because they are only interested in the diagnosis. Knowing he is facing the possibility of heart surgery, I imagine he would be feeling some degree of apprehension. This adds another layer of meaning to his desire for students to show courage when they have to examine a stranger. He may be disappointed that they don't try to understand and empathise with him, as he has done for them.

He suggests a change that could improve his experience of these examinations: for students to ask him a few questions, 'just to get a little bit to know the person'. Patients are asked not to speak while someone is listening to their heart, because vocalisation makes it difficult to hear the sounds. Victor implies this would be acceptable, if he had an opportunity beforehand to tell something about himself; the implication is that this might diminish the objectifying effects of the examination.

In stark contrast to his previous light-hearted tone, when Victor tells me about feeling treated 'like a dummy' he speaks loudly and emphatically, sounding frustrated. He regrets the students' lack of interest in his experience, sounding disheartened when he refers to their lack of emotional connection: 'Doesn't look like they feel – or have that human feeling for you'. The changes in tone during his storytelling performance in the research interview can be interpreted as embodying the emotions he has felt during his experiences of objectification.

It was Victor's own treating doctor who led the tutorial and asked Victor to allow the student to examine him. This is likely to have provided an additional motivation for him to participate: to accommodate the doctor's request in return for the help he had received. His positive relationship with the doctor may account for the fact that he is not at all critical of his role in the tutorial. He may have been unaware that the doctor might have instructed the student not to converse with him and did not realise that he could have altered the interaction in a number of ways. For example, the doctor could have cut short the process when it took longer than expected or checked how Victor was feeling and whether he wanted to continue. Patients in hospital are often expected to maintain a positive demeanour, and the expression of negative emotions can be discouraged (Sweet & Wilson, 2011). My interview with Victor provided an opportunity for him to express his frustration and disappointment by focusing on this aspect of his experience of being examined by students.

During the tutorial, Victor had little or no opportunity for identity construction, but in the research interview, he does so by telling this story, which exposes the complexity of the tutorial encounter. Victor portrays himself as an active agent by expressing empathy for students and critically evaluating them, identifying himself as an altruistic and empathic adult, like a parent or a teacher. This is juxtaposed with his account of being treated like a passive object.

I can only speculate as to why Victor closed his eyes for several minutes during the examination, because I failed to ask him about it. Some patients choose to avert their gaze during physical examinations, especially those of an intimate nature (Robinson, 2006). This may be a way of managing embarrassment when a physical examination produces 'contradictory demands of being a person and an object' (Meerabeau, 1999, p. 1510). Medical practice has developed rituals through which activities that would be socially unacceptable in other circumstances become normalised. Despite this, a physical examination can be an ambiguous experience for both examiner and patient. It can be difficult to maintain a distinction between medical and non-medical interpretations of a given situation (Meerabeau, 1999). Where there is close and prolonged physical proximity, such as when the student leaned over Victor's chest to listen to his heart, closing his eyes may have reduced Victor's discomfort. It is interesting that Brian, the patient whose story is told in Chapter 7, also closed his eyes for several minutes during a prolonged examination.

Objectivity and objectification

Students are encouraged to adopt an objective position in relation to patients. This can be constructive, contributing to medical knowledge by rendering body parts or processes 'external and concrete, situating them as perceptually objective' (Rice, 2008, p. 294). Unfortunately, *objectivity* is sometimes conflated with *objectification* – that is, treating a human being as an object 'and rendering [them] liable to manipulation or control' (Rice, 2008, p. 294). Students and clinical teachers will be better able to avoid treating a person as a non-human object if they are aware of the distinction between objectivity and objectification.

In an ethnographic study into how students learn to listen to the heart, patients with abnormal heart sounds reported feeling that students related to them as a kind of curiosity (Rice, 2008). They were in a similar situation to Victor – highly sought after for examinations because they had unusual murmurs. Typically, the examination of the heart is carried out without asking the patient any questions, especially when the focus is on making the diagnosis from the sounds alone. Many patients felt their individuality was disregarded in these interactions and the experience of objectification was distinctly negative. One said being examined felt like 'an invasion of privacy ... dehumanizing ... like you're a leaf under a microscope' (Rice, 2008, p. 303). Later, the same patient explained that she had eventually become more relaxed about being examined and that her condition had only been discovered because someone had listened to her heart, enabling her to receive timely treatment. Like Robin and Victor, her gratitude and altruism towards future patients led her to tolerate the unpleasant aspects of the examination.

Demonstrating the signs

The final story in this chapter tells about an interaction I observed on a neurosurgical ward round. Although there was no direct interaction between the patient and the medical students, the incident only happened because students were present. The patient was unable to tell her own story, because she had lost the power of speech. I believe that as an ethnographer, I have a responsibility to tell the stories of those who are unable to speak for themselves (Bosk, 1992; Denzin, 1997).

The ward round took place between 7:00 and 8:00 am and was the time for registrars (trainee surgeons) and other members of the treating team to review patients before the morning's operating session. It could also be an opportunity for the impromptu teaching of students. Time was short, so only a few minutes were spent with each patient and there was little direct communication with them. As others have described in the context of ward rounds, most interactions took place between staff as they stood around the bed (Sweet & Wilson, 2011). There were few introductions, and permission was not sought for students to be present. This applied to my own presence as well, although I had asked the doctor to seek permission from patients for me to be there.

About halfway through the round, the registrar approached an elderly lady lying in bed, and asked her how she was. When she did not answer, the senior nurse in charge of the ward told him that Mrs White was unable to speak after her recent stroke. The doctor then addressed the students, saying: 'Have you ever seen frontal lobe signs?' He began to demonstrate the signs on the woman's body, tapping her lips to elicit reflex pouting, tracing along her palm to produce a grasp, and tapping her forehead to produce blinking. While he did this, the patient put her left arm out as if to ward him off and her face developed a pained expression. The doctor continued with his demonstration, ignoring her non-verbal protest. There was no response from those watching to the indications that the patient found the examination unwelcome. When he had finished, the senior nurse reminded him that Mrs White's relatives were still waiting to meet with him to discuss her condition.

Power, identity and customary practice

When Mrs White did not respond to the doctor's initial question, he made no further attempts to communicate, and his subsequent actions suggested that he saw her as a convenient object for teaching. He did not seek her consent to him using her body in this way. His failure to acknowledge her non-verbal responses was consistent with his identification of her as an object, not as a person with individuality, agency and emotions. Through this act, he reinforced his position of power and the patient's vulnerability, restricting her already limited ability to perform her identity. This is another manifestation of the connection between relations of power and identity that was explored in the previous chapter. In contrast with the doctor's objectifying treatment, the nurse's remarks identified this patient as a person by using her name, reminding him of her loss of speech and relaying her family's concerns.

A number of factors may have contributed to this doctor's actions. He was under time pressure because established work practices required him to see all the patients before arriving on time at the operating theatre. The presence of the students would have motivated him to act like a teacher and show them this patient's signs. As the senior doctor on the round, he was in a powerful position, and even though the senior nurse drew his attention to the patient as a person, his actions went otherwise unchallenged. Although he might have been dismayed to know that his actions were interpreted as dehumanising, the doctor gave no indication that he considered her permission should have been sought before using her as an object for teaching. It is likely that he had observed similar behaviour from superiors, so that it had become consistent with his professional identity.

In a book exploring ethically important moments in health care, ethicist and university academic Lynn Gillam told of a personal experience many years earlier that had stayed in her memory (Guillemin & Gillam, 2006). She was attending a hospital outpatient clinic for investigation of rectal bleeding. A young doctor examined her and left the room, returning with a surgeon and a group of students. While she was still lying on the couch facing the wall, each of them was invited by the surgeon to look at her rectum through a rigid metal instrument called a sigmoidoscope, without her consent. It was uncomfortable and embarrassing, and she felt unable to express her objections. When one student asked if it was OK, she said yes, despite desperately wanting it to stop. She was so distressed afterwards that she had to wait some time to regain her composure before being able to drive home. Gillam's story illustrates the limits of consent in situations of vulnerability and is another example of objectification in everyday clinical practice. It also highlights the power relations operating in a teaching hospital, even for individuals with considerable status in other contexts.

Dehumanisation and dissonance

When patients are involved only as passive material on which students learn, and are prevented from telling their stories, this can intensify their sense of being treated as a non-human object. Dehumanisation occurs when an individual or group is treated as though they lack human qualities, needs or emotions. Unfortunately, there are many instances of dehumanisation in social interactions, for example between people identifying with different ethnic, racial or religious groups. They also take place in clinical encounters, including interactions involving medical students (Haslam, 2007; Rice, 2008).

Students and junior doctors often report that they have seen doctors interact with patients in ways they consider derogatory or unethical (Comstock & Williams, 1980; Dyrbye, Thomas, & Shanafelt, 2005; Gaufberg, Batalden, Sands, & Bell, 2010). One study concluded that it was common for students to see patients 'stripped of their uniqueness (stories, personality, culture) in service to objectivity' (Gaufberg et al., 2010, p. 1711). Those in subordinate positions in the hospital hierarchy often feel unable to object when patients are treated in this way and may even find themselves colluding with the behaviour. When they are expected to act in ways that are inconsistent with the values of their long-established identities, a distressing sense of internal conflict, described as *identity dissonance* can arise, with potential negative effects on their well-being (Dyrbye et al., 2005; Goldie, 2012; Monrouxe, 2010).

Most ambulatory patients participating in a study into their experiences of having medical students present during their consultations reported that the impact was either neutral or positive (McLachlan et al., 2012). They described their involvement as mainly passive, and they were not drawn into the community of practice constituted by the doctor and student, who mainly interacted with each other. Although some patients were content to be used as an object for learning, others experienced it as embarrassing and unwanted, especially when an examination of an intimate area was involved. One participant put it this way: 'They're never going to hear your story because it isn't coming across in the interview … It does make the feeling of alienation worse … and you're not involved, you are an object in those situations' (McLachlan et al., 2012, p. 969). She went on to say that she felt as though something had been taken from her. In contrast, when she had an opportunity to participate more actively, she gained satisfaction from helping students learn.

Victor's reflections on the importance of being able to tell his story echo those of this participant. Both Robin and Victor indicated they would be willing to be involved in students' learning again. Robin insisted he did not mind being used as a passive object, although he felt more positive about his involvement when he was engaged as an active participant. Having an opportunity to tell their stories, and therefore to construct and perform their identities, is clearly very important to some patients, but perhaps less so to others. Clinical teachers need to be sensitive to individual patient's needs and circumstances when considering whether and how to involve them in students' learning (McLachlan et al., 2012). Patients who are invited to participate should be given a careful explanation of what would be required of them, as well as debriefing afterwards and resolution of any concerns raised. Clinical teachers and students should always speak about patients' condition with them in terms they can understand rather than about them to others, in their presence (Chretien et al., 2010; Fletcher, Rankey, & Stern, 2005; Nair et al., 1997; Romano, 1941).

A movement has been proposed towards a *triadic* model of medical education, linking patient, student and doctor, in which the patient has an active role and the doctor acts as expert resource (Bleakley & Bligh, 2008). A number of strategies have been recommended to promote more active and inclusive patient involvement. This may include arranging for a student to interview the patient before he or she sees the doctor, placing furniture to allow more of a three-way interaction or promoting talk between the student and patient during the main consultation (McLachlan et al., 2012).

Dehumanisation in everyday practice

Two forms of dehumanisation can be distinguished, both of which involve the denial of human qualities to other people (Haslam, 2006). The first is often associated with relationships between different nations or ethnic groups and involves representing the other as a non-human animal. The second form, commonly associated with clinical interactions, involves treating others as objects that lack human qualities such as emotion, warmth, agency and individuality (Haslam, 2006). This is similar to the concept of objectification (Rice, 2008).

Several stories in this chapter depict encounters in which people are dehumanised or objectified. Students and junior doctors commonly report witnessing or participating in this type of interaction (Comstock & Williams, 1980; Gaufberg et al., 2010). Robin has the impression that students think of him as a 'piece of equipment' and are not interested in his experience. He prefers being involved in students' learning in ways that allow him to feel like an active collaborator. Victor also laments their apparent lack of emotional concern.

Dehumanisation is an everyday social phenomenon which denies a person's individual identity, and also their membership of a community of people caring for one another (Haslam, 2006, p. 252). It can be understood as a form of moral exclusion, through which people 'are placed outside the boundary in which moral values, rules and considerations of fairness apply' (Haslam, 2006, p. 254). Other forms of moral exclusion include condescension, treating others as if they were non-existent, and an exclusive focus on technical matters and routines. Stripped of agency and a sense of common humanity, the other person may 'lose the capacity to evoke compassion and moral emotions', making it easier for people to treat them as a means to serve their own ends (Haslam, 2006, p. 254). There is an associated inability to identify with that person, and a lack of empathic distress when they are treated in ways that would otherwise be socially unacceptable (Haslam, 2006). The behaviour of the registrar towards Mrs White, the patient with frontal lobe signs, can be framed in this way, as can that of the surgeon towards Lynn Gillam in her story about the rectal examination (Guillemin & Gillam, 2006).

There is an important connection between students' emotionally disturbing experiences of identity dissonance, and empathy decline and dehumanisation (Haslam, 2006, 2007; Monrouxe, 2010; Goldie, 2012). Developing empathy – learning to appreciate another's emotions and to communicate that understanding to them – is an effective way to counteract dehumanisation (Haslam, 2007). There is considerable evidence of a tendency to develop cynical and dehumanising attitudes and behaviour over time during medical training, which may be associated with a reduction in the capacity for empathy (Feudtner et al., 1994; Bleakley, 2005; Montgomery, 2006; Crandall & Marion, 2009; Hojat et al., 2009). There is both direct and indirect evidence of improved health outcomes for patients when doctors are perceived as being more empathic (Haslam, 2007; Hojat et al., 2011).

In its Code of Conduct for Good Medical Practice in Australia, the profession affirms that a key responsibility is 'to protect and promote the health of individuals and the community' (Australian Medical Council, 2014, p. 5). Good practice also 'involves doctors understanding that each patient is unique, and working in partnership' with them (Australian Medical Council, 2014, p. 5). When medical professionals use their powerful position to relate to patients as if they were non-human objects, the values they enact are in conflict with those articulated in the Code of Practice, which specifically mandates the need for informed consent before involving patients in teaching.

In the context of organisations or health care systems, many factors can influence the way individuals conduct themselves (Frank, 2002; Hayes, 1960). Power relations in hierarchical social structures, cultural values expressed in customary practices, limited resources and the educational needs of students generate circumstances in which patients' interests are subordinated to those of the health professional or student. Although students are active agents in the construction of their identities, repeatedly observing or participating in dehumanising interactions during their clinical education is likely to influence their emerging identities. Students learn that such behaviour is compatible with their professional identity, even if they would find it unacceptable in other spheres of life.

An ethnographic study in a paediatric hospital explored how medical students used language to construct patient roles and their associated professional identities (Schrewe, Bates, Pratt, Ruitenberg, & McKellin, 2017). The use of language in such contexts entails 'a progressive and pervasive adoption of sociocultural beliefs that lead one to talk, listen, relate and act' in ways that are deemed appropriate to the profession (Schrewe et al., 2017, p. 658). Through discourse analysis, the authors identified three discourses used to talk about patients: *patient-as-disease-category*, *patient-as-educational-commodity* and *patient-as-marginalised-actor*. While acknowledging the potential benefits from employing these discourses in learning and patient care, they argue that we need to recognise the powerful impact they can have on learners and their relationships with patients in order to 'better understand how the discursive category of *patient* may be untethered from the *person* embodying it' (Schrewe et al., 2017, p. 666).

Literature on dehumanisation indicates that it is common in medical encounters for a person to be treated as if they lack human attributes such as emotion, intentionality or agency (Haslam, 2006). Competing interests and priorities and the persistence of culturally accepted practices contribute to some patients being treated in dehumanising ways during clinical teaching encounters. As well as acknowledging their experiences, focusing on these stories enables us to identify contexts or practices that may be more likely to result in a sense of objectification. Although active involvement has long been advocated, the majority of patient participation in medical education continues to be passive (Rees et al., 2007). When patients are actively involved in students' learning, this can effectively include them in the community of practice, as well as the students (Lave & Wenger, 1991). This can foster mutual learning and reciprocal benefit, unlike situations in which a patient feels something has been taken from them, and nothing given in return (McLachlan et al., 2012).

Towards active participation

There are a number of potential benefits for patients from participating in students' learning. They may learn something about their condition, enjoy the social contact or gain satisfaction from helping students (Chretien et al., 2010; McLachlan et al., 2012; Rice, 2008). All the patients I interviewed said they would agree to see students again, despite some unpleasant experiences. However, many of them reported feeling used as an object devoid of human qualities; in other words, they experienced objectification or dehumanisation.

One way to counteract the tendency for patients involved in clinical teaching to feel objectified is to involve them as active participants rather than passive objects (Bleakley & Bligh, 2008; Chur-Hansen & Koopowitz, 2004; McLachlan et al., 2012; Rees, Knight, & Wilkinson, 2007; Towle et al., 2010). Programmes featuring patients as teachers of clinical skills have been described since the 1970's, although it has been argued that the increasing popularity of simulated patients has eclipsed the active role of genuine patients (Towle et al., 2010).

People with experience of illness or disability can participate in health professionals' education in a variety of ways. This usually involves direct participation in teaching or assessment, either during everyday medical encounters, in tutorials or as trained *patient-educators* (Lauckner, Doucet, & Wells, 2012; McLachlan et al., 2012). In a number of countries, *teaching associates* are trained and employed as instructors for students and junior doctors learning to perform gynaecological, genital or rectal examinations (Coldicott, Pope, & Roberts, 2003, p. 68; Hendrickx et al., 2006; Towle et al., 2010). After appropriate training, teaching associates invite learners to perform these intimate examinations on them as part of their education programmes, providing feedback about their experience.

Less commonly, people with relevant conditions may be invited by faculty members to participate in curriculum development (Towle et al., 2010). In a collaborative partnership, one patient's story about her psychiatric illness was incorporated into a problem-based learning case (Chur-Hansen & Koopowitz, 2004). More active patient involvement has the potential to benefit all concerned. However, any changes need to be carefully planned and monitored to ensure they do not have unintended negative consequences (Towle et al., 2010).

For some years, arguments have been put forward for a more patient-centred model of medical education, in which students learn *from* and *with* patients rather than just *on* or *about* them (Bleakley & Bligh, 2008). As discussed in the first chapter of this book, situated learning theory offers a useful way of thinking about identity construction in occupational contexts (Lave & Wenger, 1991; Wenger, 1998; Rees et al., 2007). The model of legitimate peripheral participation can be applied to patients as well as students, when they are engaged actively in the teaching activity (Rees et al., 2007). Learners within a community of practice move from peripheral to full participation by engaging in hands-on activity (Lave & Wenger, 1991; Rees et al., 2007). Power relations and identity formation are critical elements in this process, and participants often assume multiple identities simultaneously, which may present competing demands. A student may be a learner but also provide care, whereas a patient may be a teacher as well as a recipient of care (Rees et al., 2007). Research into the involvement of patients in medical education raises important issues including 'power relationships, occupational culture, professionalization, role ambiguity and partnership' (Rees, Ajjawi, & Monrouxe, 2013; Rees et al., 2007, p. 361).

In their formal teaching, students are told to ensure that patients' consent is always informed and freely given. However, during my observations on the wards and in clinics and my interviews with participants, I found that this advice was often disregarded. In the next chapter, with the aid of relevant stories, I explore how students gain access to patients to learn about clinical care-related activities such as ward rounds and procedures. These stories raise troubling ethical issues and allow further exploration of relational identity construction in the context of clinical teaching, including the construction of the patient as adversary.

References

Australian Medical Council. (2014). *Good medical practice – a code of conduct for doctors in Australia* (pp. 1–25). Medical Board of Australia. Retrieved from: www.medicalboard.gov.au/Codes-Guidelines-Policies/Code-of-conduct.aspx

Bleakley, A. (2005). Stories as data, data as stories: Making sense of narrative inquiry in clinical education. *Medical Education, 39*(5), 534–540.

Bleakley, A., & Bligh, J. (2008). Students learning from patients: Let's get real in medical education. *Advances in Health Sciences Education, 13*, 89–107.

Bosk, C. (1992). *All God's mistakes: Genetic counselling in a pediatric hospital.* Chicago, IL: The University of Chicago Press.

Chretien, K., Goldman, E., Craven, K., & Faselis, C. (2010). A qualitative study of the meaning of physical examination teaching for patients. *Journal of General Internal Medicine, 25*(8), 786–791.

Chur-Hansen, A., & Koopowitz, L. (2004). The patient's voice in a problem-based learning case. *Australasian Psychiatry, 12*(1), 31–35.

Coldicott, Y., Pope, C., & Roberts, C. (2003). The ethics of intimate examination. *British Medical Journal, 326*, 97–101.

Comstock, L. M., & Williams, R. C. (1980). The way we teach ... students to care for patients. *Medical Teacher, 2*(4), 168–170.

Crandall, S., & Marion, G. (2009). Identifying attitudes towards empathy: An essential feature of professionalism. *Academic Medicine, 84*(9), 1174–1176.

Denzin, N. (1997). *Interpretive ethnography: Ethnographic practices for the 21st century.* Thousand Oaks, CA: Sage.

Dyrbye, L., Thomas, M., & Shanafelt, T. (2005). Medical student distress: Causes, consequences and proposed solutions. *Mayo Clinic Proceedings, 80*(12), 1613–1622.

Feudtner, C., Christakis, D., & Christakis, N. (1994). Do clinical clerks suffer ethical erosion? Students' perceptions of their ethical environment and personal development. *Academic Medicine, 69*(8), 670–679.

Fletcher, K., Furney, S., & Stern, D. (2007). Patients speak: What's really important about bedside interactions with physician teams. *Teaching and Learning in Medicine, 19*(2), 120–127.

Fletcher, K., Rankey, D., & Stern, D. (2005). Bedside interactions from the other side of the bedrail. *Journal of General Internal Medicine, 20*, 58–61.

Frank, A. W. (2002). 'How can they act like that?' Physicians and patients as characters in each other's stories. *Hastings Center Report, 32*(6), 14–22.

Gaufberg, E., Batalden, M., Sands, R., & Bell, S. (2010). The hidden curriculum: What can we learn from third-year medical student narrative reflections? *Academic Medicine, 85*, 1709–1716.

Goldie, J. (2012). The formation of professional identity in medical students: Considerations for educators. *Medical Teacher, 34*, e641–e648.

Guillemin, M., & Gillam, L. (2006). *Telling moments: Everyday ethics in health care.* Melbourne: IP Communications.

Haslam, N. (2006). Dehumanization: An integrative review. *Personality and Social Psychology Review, 10*(3), 252–264.

Haslam, N. (2007). Humanising medical practice: The role of empathy. *Medical Journal of Australia, 187*(7), 381–382.

Hayes, G. (1960). The patient looks at the medical school hospital. *Journal of the American Medical Association, 173*(12), 1305–1307.

Hendrickx, K., De Winter, B. Y., Wyndaele, J.-J., Tjalma, W. A. A., Debaene, L., Selleslags, B., ... Bossaert, L. (2006). Intimate examination teaching with volunteers: Implementation and assessment at the University of Antwerp. *Patient Education and Counseling, 63*(1–2), 47–54.

Hojat, M., Vergare, M., Maxwell, K., Brainard, G., Herrine, S., Isenberg, G., ... Gonnella, J. (2009). The devil is in the third year: A longitudinal study of erosion of empathy in medical school. *Academic Medicine, 84*(9), 1182–1191.

Hojat, M., Louis, D. Z., Markham, F. W., Wender, R., Rabinowitz, C., & Gonnella, J. S. (2011). Physicians' empathy and clinical outcomes for diabetic patients. *Academic Medicine, 86*(3), 359–364 310.1097/ACM.1090b1013e318208 6fe3182081.

Lauckner, H., Doucet, S., & Wells, S. (2012). Patients as educators: The challenges and benefits of sharing experiences with students. Medical Education, 46(10), 992–1000. doi: 10.1111/j.1365-2923.2012.04356.x

Lave, J., & Wenger, E. (1991). *Situated learning: Legitimate peripheral participation.* Cambridge: Cambridge University Press.

McLachlan, E., King, N., Wenger, E., & Dornan, T. (2012). Phenomenological analysis of patient experiences of medical student teaching encounters. *Medical Education, 46*(10), 963–973. doi:10.1111/j.1365-2923.2012.04332.x

Medical Board of Australia. (2009). *Good medical practice: A code of conduct for doctors in Australia.* (p. 19).

Meerabeau, L. (1999). The management of embarrassment and sexuality in health care. *Journal of Advanced Nursing, 29*(6), 1507–1513.

Monrouxe, L. (2010). Identity, identification and medical education: Why should we care? *Medical Education, 44*(1), 40–49. doi:10.1111/j.1365-2923.2009.03440.x

Monrouxe, L., Rees, C., & Bradley, P. (2009). The construction of patients' involvement in hospital bedside teaching encounters. *Qualitative Health Research, 19*(7), 918–930. doi:10.1177/1049732309338583

Montgomery, K. (2006). *How doctors think: Clinical judgement and the practice of medicine.* New York: Oxford University Press.

Nair, B. R., Coughlan, J. L., & Hensley, M. J. (1997). Student and patient perspectives on bedside teaching. *Medical Education, 31*, 341–346.

Rees, C., Ajjawi, R., & Monrouxe, L. V. (2013). The construction of power in family medicine bedside teaching: A video observation study. *Medical Education, 47*(2), 154–165. doi:10.1111/medu.12055

Rees, C., Knight, L. V., & Wilkinson, C. E. (2007). 'User involvement is a sine qua non, almost, in medical education': Learning with rather than just about health and social care service users. *Advances in Health Sciences Education: Theory and Practice, 12*(3), 359–390.

Rice, T. (2008). 'Beautiful murmurs': Stethoscopic listening and acoustic objectification. *The Senses and Society, 3*, 293–306. doi:10.2752/174589308X331332

Robinson, J. D. (2006). Nonverbal communication and physician-patient interaction. In V. Manusov & M. Patterson (Eds.), *The Sage handbook of nonverbal communication* (pp. 437–459). Thousand Oaks, CA: Sage.

Romano, J. (1941). Patients' attitudes and behavior in ward round teaching. *JAMA (Chicago, Ill.), 117*(9), 664–667.

Schrewe, B., Bates, J., Pratt, D., Ruitenberg, C. W., & McKellin, W. H. (2017). The Big D(eal): Professional identity through discursive constructions of 'patient'. *Medical Education, 51*(6), 656–668. doi:10.1111/medu.13299

Sweet, G. S., & Wilson, H. J. (2011). A patient's experience of ward rounds. *Patient Education and Counselling, 84*(2), 150–151. doi: 10.1016/j.pec.2010.08.016

Towle, A., Bainbridge, L., Godolphin, W., Katz, A. M., Kline, C., Lown, B., … Thistlethwaite, J. (2010). Active patient involvement in the education of health professionals. *Academic Medicine, 44*, 64–74.

Wenger, E. (1998). *Communities of practice: Learning, meaning and identity.* Cambridge: Cambridge University Press.

6 Allies and adversaries*

The patients with the conditions that you need to see ... you ask the question in such a way, you make it hard for them to say no. ... Because we're early on in the year we don't really push the issue too much, but I think, you know, if this was a patient with a rare condition that I desperately needed to see before my exam, you probably would have just pushed the issue a little bit more. ... But I think most people are happy to participate. And – you know, ultimately it's ten, 15 minutes, it's not that much. If we clearly see a patient's not up to it, we wouldn't do it. Um – and to a large extent I think, you know ... in a public hospital setting, patients if they're well – shouldn't really say no. Unless there's a particularly strong clinical reason, either they are very unwell or it's a particularly emotional situation; but your average, you know, 80, 70-year-old patient who's had a bit of chest pain or whatever, should understand that – and I think it's even spelt out in a lot of the hospital brochures that – 'You may have medical students coming to talk to you. We encourage you to agree and participate because it's important'. So, so I think that patients shouldn't really say no. Yeah. I wouldn't say no.

Robert, trainee specialist physician and tutor

Obligation or option

Robert, a young doctor and clinical tutor who recently completed his specialist examinations, acknowledges the potential conflict between the needs of patients and those of students or doctors-in-training. Specialist exams are highly demanding, and candidates are under pressure to examine as many patients as possible with unusual clinical signs. Robert says that he would put more pressure on patients when exams are imminent or when they have a rare condition. He thinks public patients should not refuse to be seen by students or trainee specialists unless they are very unwell or distressed. Perhaps to refute potential arguments against this view, he refers to hospital brochures as an authority, and states that he would not object if he were a patient.

A number of arguments have been advanced to support the view that patients have a moral obligation to participate in medical students' clinical teaching and learning activities (Waterbury, 2001). For patients receiving state-funded services, their involvement may be seen as a form of payment for services received.

Some of my student participants maintained that patients should participate because clinical training is indispensable for doctors. However, I agree with the ethical analysis of these and other arguments that any obligation to provide clinical training lies with the educational institution rather than individual patients (Waterbury, 2001).

Students' participation in the everyday work of doctors is an indispensable part of their training. In this chapter, students share stories about how they gain access to patients in ward rounds and clinics. They also tell about experiences of participating in patient care-related activities, performing simple procedures like collecting blood specimens and inserting intravenous lines. I discuss how students view these practices, consider implications for their emerging professional identities and highlight some troubling ethical issues raised by their stories.

In these stories we see how patients and doctors may come to be identified by students either as adversaries or allies, and how this can influence students' emerging professional identities. Students observe how interactions take place in the community of practice they aspire to join. Commonly accepted or *customary* practices both reveal and reproduce values that are at odds with the standards of integrity claimed by the profession and advocated in medical schools (Australian Medical Council, 2014; Medical Board of Australia, 2009; World Medical Association, 2006 [1949]).

Revealing everyday consent practices

In their introductory week, students were directed by faculty members to obtain valid consent from patients before undertaking any interview, examination or procedure. However, strategies were suggested to increase the chances of patients agreeing to see them, for example describing themselves as student doctors instead of medical students. The implication was that the resulting ambiguity could be to students' advantage.

Students must learn to appropriately perform examinations of parts of the body considered sensitive: those that are often associated with strong emotions. These include breast, genital, gynaecological and rectal examinations. The use of anatomical models can assist with the acquisition of technical skills, but the greatest challenge lies in the sensitivity of the interpersonal exchange, the mastery of which requires an authentic human encounter.

At universities in countries including the USA, Canada, Australia and the Netherlands, trained teaching associates have been engaged to help students and junior doctors learn to perform gynaecological, rectal and urogenital examinations (Hendrickx et al., 2006; Robertson, Hegarty, O'Connor, & Gunn, 2003). The involvement of patients in this role has the additional benefit of shifting the power dynamics between students and patients, creating a different kind of clinical encounter. Teachers, learners and volunteers have evaluated these programmes positively, but they are not without risk. There is the potential for teaching associates to experience discomfort or distress and this risk must be managed sensitively by programme co-ordinators (Robertson et al., 2003; Taylor, 2011).

Despite these innovations, a study of medical students in the United Kingdom found that vaginal and rectal examinations continued to be performed under anaesthesia without patients' consent (Coldicott, Pope, & Roberts, 2003). Many students felt unable to refuse a doctor's request to perform the examinations or to voice their concerns. In a later study, students from medical schools in the United Kingdom and Australia reported witnessing or being asked to perform sensitive examinations where consent had not been obtained (Rees & Monrouxe, 2011).

Many students' attitudes towards obtaining consent change over their time in medical school, diverging further from those of patients themselves. Patients place much greater importance than students do on the need to gain consent from them if a student intends to carry out a rectal examination while they are anaesthetised (Silver-Isenstadt & Ubel, 1999). The difference was greater for students in their clinical years of training; more than a quarter of those students participating in the study did not consider it important to gain consent from patients for such examinations (Silver-Isenstadt & Ubel, 1999).

When patients do not give informed consent and are not informed that the person examining them is a student, this raises a number of ethical issues. Most importantly, they cannot exercise their right to accept or refuse students' involvement. In addition, they cannot make allowances for a students' lack of skill and confidence, or gain satisfaction from the knowledge that they have been helpful (Silver-Isenstadt & Ubel, 1999). There may also be potential consequences for *students* in relation to their emerging identities and future interactions with patients, as the stories in this chapter reveal.

Talking about sensitive examinations

I attended a tutorial designed to enhance students' ability to communicate effectively with patients in challenging situations. It focused on talking with patients about the rectal examination (PR), and was led by Daniel, one of the tutors I had previously interviewed. No patients were present. The content was designed in collaboration with a communications expert, and much of it was relevant to other examinations such as the breasts or genitalia, which can also arouse difficult emotions. Daniel spoke about why you might need to do a PR, some possible findings and their interpretation. He demonstrated the technique on a plastic and rubber anatomical model and advised students how to speak with a patient before, during and after the examination. Students practised this exercise in pairs with his guidance, and all were actively engaged in the process.

In the following passage from his tutorial, Daniel explains how to seek a patient's agreement and respond to those who decline or appear reluctant.

People want to know what will happen to them. Often, we don't tell them, and it freaks them out; their anxiety goes up tremendously. If you put a finger in and they're not expecting it, they go: 'Whoa – what happened?' They might want to know what side effects there could be, like, 'Will there be any pain?' Usually it's best to say discomfort, and then they're less likely to experience pain. … We often joke to hide our own discomfort, but it's not appropriate in this situation to be flippant. You need to be as professional as possible.

If they do refuse – what should we do, if it's important? … Well, we should always explore their reasons for refusing – this is important for anything we want to do. Start by checking their understanding – do they know exactly what you want to do? Then explain why you believe it's important. But in the end, don't forget that we have to respect their choice. … You need to ask about their concerns if they seem reluctant. Say that if it hurts, they can tell you to stop. You need to empower them – let them know it's an option and that you will listen to them.

Also, you need to think about the person's cultural and personal background, and how that might affect their feelings about the examination. There are a lot of victims of sexual abuse out there. Having a PR exam can be very sensitive for them. Think about refugees, and people from groups who may have been the target of ethnic cleansing, or Holocaust survivors. … Have your antennae open to look out for these possibilities. Having said that, most people go along happily with what you want to do – well, maybe not happily, but willingly.

From my previous interview with him, I know Daniel takes the task of teaching students very seriously. During the tutorial, he identifies himself as an experienced doctor and as a result, students are likely to take notice of his advice. He demonstrates how humour can be used to deal with a taboo subject, but warns students not to be flippant when talking with a patient.

Daniel explains that a doctor can make a difficult experience worse by being insensitive to patients' needs, emphasising that they tend to feel more anxious without detailed information about what is going to happen. He reminds students that patients are entitled to decline but may need to be empowered to do so, for example by checking at every stage whether they are comfortable to proceed.

He draws students' attention to the connotations a rectal or genital examination may have for people with a history of abuse, asking them to consider how each person's history creates particular meanings for them which could differ from how the students would feel themselves in the same situation. His advice to show empathy by considering the patient's perspective contrasts with Robert's view that patients should agree to see students because he would, if he were a patient. In Bakhtinian terms, Daniel relates to the patients dialogically whereas Robert's way of relating is more monological.

Daniel invites his audience to enter into the experience of both parties, representing the doctor's experience using the language of medicine and employing lay terms that could be used to address the patient. Explaining why patients may have difficulty expressing reluctance or refusing a doctor's request, Daniel refers explicitly to the relations of power between doctor and patient. However, he does not mention the power asymmetry between doctors and students or advise students how to respond if asked to perform a sensitive examination without consent. He fails to address another issue as well: whether a patient should be explicitly offered the option to have a qualified doctor perform the examination, rather than a student.

Consent and the physical examination

Thao told this story after speaking of his disappointment that patients' emotional and social needs were often neglected, because of the great demands on the time of hospital staff. He was concerned that he might develop a cynical attitude towards patients and that constant exposure to distressed patients would affect his own well-being. I asked him to tell me about a time when he had encountered a distressed patient.

> Recently I was in a clinic and this lady had a past history of breast cancer. And so, she was just coming in for a check-up and the doctor there was – [pause] I don't want to make a generalisation, but he was a surgeon. And he was just palpating her breast and he found a lump. And [pause] usually – it's um – a normal occurrence if you get a bit of, like, scar tissue underneath the actual incision but um – the lump was slightly [pause] to the side of the scar. And so, that pretty much meant that she had a recurrence of her cancer. And when the doctor broke that news to her she started crying, and then – um – the doctor asked me to – feel the lump, except he didn't really ask the patient if there was any consent at all.

> So, what did you do?

> Um – I asked the patient if that was OK, and she said it was OK, but the doctor seemed to brush over that, I guess.

> OK, so that surprised you, that he didn't give much priority to asking [the patient] – what about the fact that she was upset? How did the doctor react to that?

> He done the usual: 'Yeah, it's bad news, but we're not too sure yet'. Umm – [pause] he didn't really take it into account I guess [rising inflection, suggesting uncertainty]. He was polite but he didn't actually acknowledge the actual feeling that she had. ... He didn't offer a tissue or anything at all. ... And, he just went on with – [pause] work, I guess.

> And then – so you're feeling the lump; were you able to say anything? Or it wasn't really possible.

> I don't think it was that possible. Yeah.

> So you felt –

> Really, really awkward. And I don't think – if I had got that type of bad news, I don't think I would want a medical student in there.

Thao tells of his discomfort at having to perform a breast exam without consent and being present when a patient was given distressing news. The consultation is originally described as routine and Thao hints at the stereotype of surgeons as insensitive. The encounter becomes anything but routine when the doctor feels a lump and explains this could indicate a cancer recurrence. To Thao's dismay, he instructs him to feel the lump without asking permission. He interprets the doctor's behaviour as indicating a lack of consideration: 'He was polite, but he didn't actually acknowledge the actual feeling that she had'. He continues with his work, possibly writing in the notes, or ordering investigations. In contrast, Thao is considering the patient's feelings and imagines how he would feel in her position: 'If I had got that type of bad news, I don't think I would want a medical student in there'.

Thao finds himself in a difficult situation. His subordinate relationship to the surgeon prevents him from directly criticising him about the lack of consent, but he asks the woman whether it would be OK for him to examine her breast. In doing so, he distances himself from the surgeon's lack of response to the woman's distress and acknowledges that she might prefer not to have a student examine her. When she says it's OK, he proceeds with the examination but continues to feel uncomfortable.

He identifies himself as compassionate but also vulnerable and disillusioned at the way many doctors relate to patients. The surgeon is characterised as uncaring and detached; he does not even offer the distressed woman a tissue. Thao's experience could be characterised as one of identity dissonance: his established identity and values conflict with the behaviour expected of him as a medical student. Repeated experiences of identity dissonance can have profound effects on some students' well-being (Monrouxe, 2010).

Patients attending a gynaecology clinic who were seen by students for the first time were more uncomfortable about it than they were on future occasions (Hartz & Beal, 2000). The extent of the student's proposed involvement should be detailed by doctors when consent is sought for them to be present. During my fieldwork, it was common for doctors in a clinic to briefly ask: 'Is it OK for a student to join us?' This made it difficult for a patient to decline or even to know what they were agreeing to. It is possible that many doctors proceed on the assumption that a patient has agreed to the student participating in anything the doctor deems appropriate. This is one potential explanation for the actions of the surgeon in Thao's story.

Consent and performing procedures

Grace told me this story when I asked her what it was like asking patients if you could perform a procedure on them.

> Consent is a bit different with procedures. A lot of the time – the doctor or the intern or resident will just quickly ask. It's usually a one sentence thing: 'So you need to get a drip put in. Is it OK if the student does it?' and then

usually the patient says 'Yes' or in some cases 'No'. I don't think I've had any patients who have said 'No' to me. But it's not unheard of, particularly if the patient has had prior experiences – which you completely understand. That being said, I do remember my one venepuncture for this man which I don't think ended up very pleasantly for him. I caused him a lot of pain, yeah, which was unfortunate.

Did you need to have more than one go, or –?

Well, my rule is that I don't have a second go on a patient. I'm not going to try twice. If I've caused – if I've failed the first time, I'll let someone who's actually had experience do it. But – um – this man, I think I wasn't very confident and so my technique wasn't very good, and I think I just put it too shallowly, and that causes a lot of pain … which isn't very good, and the intern did take over. I did actually manage to get it signed off [in the log book], because I think I got blood in the end, [both laugh] but it wasn't a particularly good experience for the patient, and in those cases I think even if it is successful it can be marred by the patient's experience of it. That being said, there are other times, like when I put a drip in this man's arm, and I think he was on so many drugs that he just didn't feel anything. That being said, he bled so much, like just over – it was on my gloves and over that blue mattress thing. I was completely freaking out, but the patient was fine.

Was there someone supervising?

Oh yes, definitely. … I wouldn't do it without supervision. I have been asked to do it without supervision in the past. But I've chosen not to. I don't have that much confidence in my skills.

And do you think the patient knows that they could say 'No'? Or is it sort of presented as though 'This is what's going to happen'?

I think with procedures – it's a bit easier for the patient to understand why we need to practise just because – it's a procedural skill and you can't quite learn it out of a textbook. And I think that's how we approach it as well. Procedural skills just have to be done … and so – we – feel – less guilty – with – um – um – not – a hundred per cent consenting the patient as we should, and as we've been taught in the past – of um – you know, who we are, why we're doing it and things like that. We're happy to just do it on a patient even though they're not quite aware if we're a student or if we're practising.

And do you get an impression that doctors … think patients should let students do procedures on them?

I think doctors are more on the side of the students when it comes to these things just because I think they have been students in the past and they've gone through the same thing. … In most cases they'll try to push for – not push, but they'll just ask on behalf of you and often because they're the doctor, then the patient will agree. … And that's not to say that the doctor isn't aware of the patient's, maybe, misgivings. I think we're <u>all</u> aware, [laughs] on some level, that the patient might not be a hundred per cent happy that we're doing this. But we do it anyway, for the reasons that I've given, particularly for procedural skills.

In this passage, Grace talks about the difference between obtaining consent to practise procedures on patients and the protocols students are taught in the formal curriculum. She describes two experiences of taking blood: one which caused a patient pain, and another which distressed <u>her,</u> but did not seem to bother the patient. She asserts that she would never do a procedure without supervision, despite having been asked to do so, and would not have a second try after an unsuccessful attempt. She argues that customary practices of obtaining consent are justified because if valid processes were followed, students might not gain sufficient practice to become proficient at procedures.

Grace's story shows that there is a risk of patients experiencing additional pain or distress from students performing procedures, even when supervised. When I enquire what it's like asking patients about performing procedures, Grace pauses and laughs, saying that 'consent is a bit different for procedures' before describing how it is done. These non-verbal elements of Grace's performance imply that she is uncomfortable about what she is about to say. Later, she hesitates seven times in a sequence of ten words: 'so – we – feel – less guilty – with – um – um – not – a hundred per cent consenting the patient as we should'. This suggests she is unsure about how to express what she feels, or reluctant to

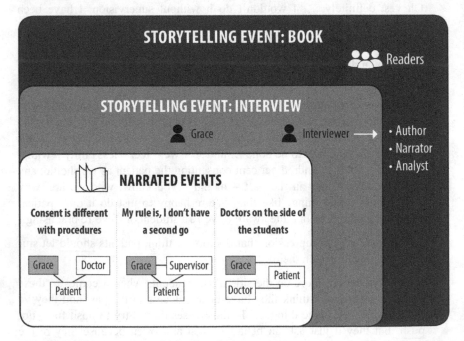

Figure 6.1 Grace's story: multi-level analysis.

admit to not obtaining valid consent as she has been taught. The plural pronoun 'we' can have the effect of abrogating responsibility; in this case, it also implies that her actions are consistent with those of her peers and supervising doctors (Rees & Monrouxe, 2008, p. 179).

Grace refers to *consenting the patient* rather than *obtaining consent from the patient*. During my fieldwork, I often heard students use this expression, and one student criticised an ethics lecturer who had denounced it, insisting it was just a convenient abbreviation. This expression is troubling because it represents consent as something *done to* rather than *given by* the patient. It characterises the patient as passive, and further enhances the agency of the doctor or student doing the 'consenting'. When I ask whether patients know they could decline, Grace remarks that it is 'easier for the patient to understand why we need to practise'. However, she then argues that it is acceptable for students to perform procedures on patients without fully informing them, which seems inconsistent with her claim that patients understand why they need to practise. This suggests she may have some ambivalence about these customary practices, even though she explicitly condones them.

When I ask about doctors' attitudes to whether patients should be given a choice, Grace says doctors are 'more on the side of the students', implying that doctors prioritise students' needs over those of patients. She changes her initial characterisation of doctors' approach from 'push' to 'just ask', suggesting that she wants to avoid them being seen as coercive. Her initial choice of words echoes Robert's expression 'pushing the issue' in relation to approaching patients with highly sought-after signs. This implies that she considers a degree of coercion is acceptable in some situations.

As the passage draws to a close, Grace uses a double negative: 'that's not to say the doctor isn't aware' and the hedge 'maybe' to refer to patients' misgivings. This downplays any implication that she is critical of the doctors' practices. Although she appears to be evaluating their approach positively, she highlights her refusal to comply with a request to perform an unsupervised procedure. She explains that she has maintained her own capacity to judge what is appropriate and is not merely conforming with their expectations, saying: 'I have been asked to do it without supervision in the past, but I've chosen not to'. She responds to my question about whether she needed more than one attempt on the patient in her first story by saying 'well my rule is, I don't have a second go on a patient'. The first-person singular pronouns 'my' and 'I' highlight her own agency (Rees & Monrouxe, 2008). Grace identifies herself as a person who seeks to limit the suffering patients might feel because of her inexperience.

Fear and desire have the capacity to animate, or breathe life into a story; they can be seen as complementary to each other (Frank, 2010). Desires and fears remind us of identity's material aspects, arising from the needs and vulnerabilities of our bodies (Lemke, 2008). Grace's linkage of the statement that procedures 'just have to be done' with her acknowledgement that 'we do it anyway' even when patients are reluctant, implies a fear that fully informed patients would decline to participate. The other side of this fear is the desire to gain sufficient experience to complete the year and master the necessary skills. The stories Grace tells about her experiences convey a sense of danger, indicating that procedures can arouse apprehension because of the risk of pain or distress. The complementary desire is that she will carry out a successful procedure, which does not result in suffering for either party.

Considerable identity work is accomplished by these stories. Grace positions herself in relation to patients, doctors and other students by using linguistic and performative devices and making claims and supporting arguments. She chooses stories about particular episodes that highlight the experiential nature of her knowledge. The analysis demonstrates how power relations and local practices of teaching and learning influence her emerging identity.

Consent and ward rounds

During my interview with another student, Natalie, the following story emerged when I asked whether any patients had said 'No' to seeing her. Although told as an experience of rejection, the story also addresses patient expectations and customary practices around consent in the context of ward rounds.

> I did have another experience where a patient said 'no', and it was amaz-
> ingly on a ward round; and we've never been asked to leave a ward round
> before, especially not by a patient. And we just saw this patient and it was
> quite an assertive registrar that was leading the ward round. And he wasn't
> asking any personal questions; we didn't quite understand the reason for her
> behaviour. Um – and she was … almost ready to be discharged, a lower
> level of nursing, um – and she just went, you know, 'Who are all these
> people? I don't want them here', and he was very much saying 'They're
> part of my team' – um – and she ended up demanding that we leave, and so
> we left but – but it was really nice that he was sort of representing us and
> advocating for us that we stay, and that it is a teaching hospital and um
> yeah, that was – hard to understand where that was coming from.

> I've noticed on ward rounds I've been on, they often don't say that – they
> don't always say that they're students.

> That's right. [Whispered] Yeah.

> When you say, 'it's a teaching hospital', do you think that they – should be
> required to have students there?

> I was under the impression that – um – [pause] sorry, I know – ward rounds
> were actually created, historically I think, for teaching purposes, was my
> understanding. That it – not only is it the most efficient way to review every
> patient every day, but that the consultant would teach the registrar, the reg-
> istrar would teach the intern – um – and I – I don't know, I'd never seen a
> patient exercise the right before, to demand that we leave. Um – yeah, and
> we were all pretty disappointed at that.

Did you feel that was an unreasonable thing?

I did. For a ward round – I can understand if it was a procedure, or – um – a really personal – we've been asked by the doctors to leave ward rounds before if they were seeing a palliative patient or – um – breaking news about cancer to a patient's family or that type of thing. But we'd never before been asked to leave a ward round – and most doctors would never give patients the option, and don't introduce us as students.

So, does that suggest that the doctors think that patients really ought to be seeing students, or having them present?

I think so. Yeah. And I think they probably realise that it's not helpful – to be giving patients the option not to see –

It's not helpful?

I think they realise that if you always gave patients the option not to see students that the students probably would miss out on a lot more than they already do.

Right. Suggesting that patients probably – if they knew they had a choice, they would probably prefer not.

Yeah, they might, yeah. When I think, ward rounds are not – I don't know, I'm not sure, I don't think there's anything overly personal or – the majority of our ward rounds are not highly sensitive information or emotional times; it's reviewing, you know, drug charts and fluid input and output and – whatever, yeah.

The immediate context of this narrated event is a medical ward round, but the broader context is one in which increasing numbers of students need to gain exposure to hospital patients for their clinical training, to pass their exams and prepare for their future work. The availability of suitable patients for teaching is a problem because patients in hospital tend to be more acutely unwell than in the past, and stay for a shorter time. In this case, the interaction is expected to be routine, so the patient's request to have students leave the room comes as more of a surprise than if she had been earlier in her admission.

When she objects to the students' presence, the doctor tries to persuade her to let them stay, but she insists, and the students eventually withdraw. Natalie incorporates direct speech in her story, representing the patient as saying: 'Who are all these people? I don't want them here' and the doctor: 'They're part of my team'. Through ventriloquation, by placing these expressions into the mouths of the speakers, the narrator voices the patient's behaviour as unjustified, and that of the doctor as reasonable. The words chosen to describe their actions portray the doctor in a more positive light: he 'advocates' for the students, whereas the patient 'demands' that they leave.

When I ask whether she thinks patients should be required to have students present, Natalie avoids answering directly. She refers to the historical origins of

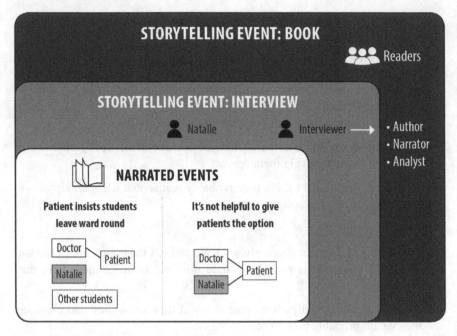

Figure 6.2 Natalie's story: multi-level analysis.

ward rounds and their teaching function to defend the consent practices she has observed. Strikingly, she drops her otherwise confident voice to a whisper as she agrees that patients are often not told of students' presence. This part of her performance suggests either that she had not previously thought about the implications of this practice, or that she thinks it should be kept quiet. Natalie has learnt that withholding information from a patient about a student's presence is acceptable, and this is likely to influence her emerging professional identity.

She is surprised to see this patient exercise her right to say 'No', implying that she believes patients need not be informed about students' presence, nor their permission sought. She supports her contention on two grounds: that nothing personal or sensitive was going to be discussed on this occasion, and that if patients were given the option, 'students probably would miss out on a lot more than they already do'. By positioning herself as supportive of the doctor's actions and opposed to those of the patient, Natalie identifies the patient as an adversary and the doctor as an ally. Her story also portrays the patient as transgressive because she fails to submit to the doctor's authority. There is also an implication that the agenda for the interaction would be determined by the doctor alone; in fact, there is no way to know what the patient herself might have wanted to talk about.

My participation in this story's production consists mainly of prompting Natalie to think about a patient who said 'No', seeking clarification of events and her evaluation of them. However, at one point I interrupt her, repeating her words 'it's not helpful?' in a challenging tone. I realise on listening to the audio recording that this was disrespectful, and that my obvious disapproval might have caused her to censor or moderate the expression of her views. Yet despite my interruption, she continues to argue in favour of the doctor's approach.

Negotiating identity in practice

Developing identity as a member of a community of practice involves learning how people in that community are expected to treat and interact with each other (Wenger, 1998). Despite individual differences, members of any social group tend to develop common perspectives, values and interpretations of events. Through sustained engagement with an occupational context, such as a teaching hospital, newcomers develop the ability to interpret and use the repertoire which full members command. 'In practice, we know who we are by what is familiar, understandable and negotiable' (Wenger, 1998, p. 153).

I use the term *practice* to indicate that there is a 'historical and social context that gives structure and meaning' to what is done, so that it is always both social and negotiated (Wenger, 1998, p. 47). Alongside what is explicitly taught, newcomers tacitly learn a vast array of conventions and rules which guide interpretation and action in that context; however, these are rarely articulated. Their incorporation into an individual's repertoire is one way in which membership of a community of practice becomes apparent.

In the stories told by Grace and Natalie about their personal experiences, certain ways of treating patients that I consider to be ethically troubling or even misleading are represented as acceptable. They include the deliberate withholding of information about a student's presence and the use of a doctor's authority to secure patients' participation. During my interview with Thao, he told me he felt that doctors sometimes used coercion to get patients to allow a student to carry out a procedure on them. Robert also implies this when he says that, if he thinks it is justified, he will ask a patient in a way that 'makes it hard to say no'.

During several interviews, when I drew attention to practices which participants had come to take for granted, their speech became hesitant as they spoke about what was usually done and attempted to justify it. This was striking in my interview with Grace, who paused seven times in the space of ten words as she admitted to not undertaking the procedures for gaining consent that she had been taught. When Natalie whispered 'that's right' after I remarked that students' presence on ward rounds was often not disclosed to patients, her tone suggested that she had not been consciously aware of this practice. This is consistent with the notion that with immersion and participation in a community of practice, its common ways of interacting and interpreting events become part of the identity which develops for newcomers (Wenger, 1998).

Grace and Natalie's reluctance to criticise the ethically troubling practices that come up during our interviews can also be considered in relation to the research on different modes of identification with social groups (Roccas, Sagiv, Schwartz, Halevy, & Eidelson, 2008). As discussed earlier, individuals have different patterns of identification with their social groups, and groups themselves may require certain modes of identification from members. Some social groups require members to identify predominantly through *glorification* (considering the group superior to others and deferring to its norms) as opposed to *attachment* (considering the group's importance to members and their desire to benefit the group). Identifying predominantly through glorification can lead members – or aspiring members in the case of medical students – to support arguments that justify group members contravening accepted moral standards. Those whose mode of identification with a given group is predominantly through attachment may be more willing to criticise members of the group if they consider their actions violate the group's values.

Negotiation, accommodation and resistance

Although students' emerging identities are heavily influenced by customary practices, identity construction is not a passive process. Students are 'active subjects who make choices, resist subjugation, accommodate power differentials, and ... actively craft themselves internally' during their training (Holmes, Jenks, & Stonington, 2011, p. 109; DelVecchio Good, 2011). Acts of negotiation, accommodation and resistance are part of many stories told by students about their experiences and contribute to their identity work. When the clinic surgeon asks Thao to examine a woman's breast without first seeking her agreement, his decision to ask her if it is OK can be seen as a courageous act, because it could be interpreted as drawing attention to the surgeon's omission. Also, if the patient had declined to be examined, he would have missed a valuable learning opportunity. Although he ultimately complied with the surgeon's direction, his question subtly altered the interaction by acknowledging her as a person who was entitled to accept or decline his request. The student who asks Gillam: 'Are you sure this is OK?', during her sigmoidoscopic examination (described in Chapter 5) shows courage because she risks antagonising the surgeon and her peers if they had consequently missed a learning opportunity (Guillemin & Gillam, 2006).

It could be argued in both cases that the students' interventions were futile, since the examination proceeded in each case, despite a lack of valid consent. However, meanings emerge for the narrator as well as the audience as a consequence of the fact that each story was told. In Gillam's story, she felt that her personhood was affirmed by the student's question, even though she was unable to voice her own dissent. Through his story, Thao identified himself as someone who maintained his view of the patient as a person, despite the risks to himself and the shortcomings he perceived in the doctor.

In prior research, when students told how they had responded to requests from doctors to observe or perform examinations without consent, they tended to portray themselves in a positive light (Rees & Monrouxe, 2011). However, when they complied with doctors' requests despite their misgivings, they highlighted their feelings of powerlessness. Occasionally, they told of their refusal to accede to a doctor's request, and highlighted their sense of agency (Rees & Monrouxe, 2011). When Grace responds to my question about whether she had needed more than one try at a procedure she highlights her agency when she says 'Well, <u>my</u> rule is I don't have a second go on a patient'.

Fear, desire and 'disavowed' motivations

A story can be animated by fears and desires, even when they are implicit and remain unacknowledged by the narrator (Frank, 2010). In her justification of customary consent practices, Grace alludes to some common concerns and aspirations of students and educators as she recounts her experiences of performing procedures on patients. The desire to gain experience is linked with a fear that an informed patient would not participate, and this fear appears to motivate withholding information from patients or failing to offer them options.

Patients and doctors often have difficulty understanding each other's motivations and actions. This may be related to conflicting priorities, which can be understood as the stakes they play for in the *game of life* (Frank, 2002). Bourdieu's concept of the *habitus* – the embodied habits and dispositions acquired as people develop in particular contexts – helps explain how these stakes are 'intimately tied to who they are, as corporeal beings' (Frank, 2002, p. 18). People often find their priorities difficult to articulate, precisely because they operate beneath conscious awareness. This makes it more challenging to acknowledge that others' priorities may differ from our own (Frank, 2002).

Natalie's story suggests that her emerging identity is shaped by her alignment with the values of the doctors. The stakes most valued by the doctors appear to be the efficient completion of their work tasks and being able to obtain maximal clinical experience for students. When Natalie implies that the agenda for the ward round is determined by the doctor, she characterises the patient as passive, with limited agency. This can be contrasted with Daniel's acknowledgement of patients' vulnerability and his argument that their agency should be promoted. Driven by her own unspoken fears and desires, similar to those revealed in Grace's story, Natalie appears unable to imagine those which might animate the patient's story.

The inferred motivations of students interviewed about their responses to video recordings of challenging scenarios were classified into three categories (Ginsburg, Regehr, & Lingard, 2003). The first category, *avowed* motivations, was aligned with the espoused values of the profession, such as placing a patient's comfort and safety first. The second category, *unavowed* motivations, was related to the idea that their actions could have implications for their relationships with fellow students or superiors. These motivations included obedience to supervising clinicians or allegiance to their peer group and, although not openly advocated, they were implicitly rewarded. The researchers expressed concern that these motivations could, in their future professional life, lead to a reluctance to disclose errors or speak up about troubling behaviour on the part of colleagues (Ginsburg et al., 2003).

The third category, *disavowed* motivations, related to students' self-interest, including concerns about the impact of their actions on their evaluation by supervisors, or their desire to avoid feelings of guilt. These motivations were disavowed or denied because self-interest is eschewed by the profession in favour of self-sacrifice (Ginsburg et al., 2003). Students and doctors could be made aware of the potential for their responses to challenging situations to be influenced by self-interested motivations. Being prepared to acknowledge this fact should be seen as an indication of their capacity for reflection. Teaching students to acknowledge and negotiate all three kinds of motivations has the potential to promote a professional stance which respects the needs of both patients and students (Ginsburg et al., 2003).

Constructing the patient as adversary

In the stories told by Grace and Natalie, patients are represented as adversaries, whereas the doctors are characterised as being 'on the side of the students'. In a study exploring how people conceptualise doctor-patient relationships, most people chose metaphors that highlighted their adversarial nature (Rees, Knight, & Wilkinson, 2007). Grace and Natalie's positioning of patients as adversaries during stories about customary consent practices indicates how this antagonistic view of patients' relationships with doctors or students can be incorporated into their emerging professional identities.

In contrast, Daniel argues for an approach which is respectful of every patient's right to make informed choices. His technical expertise and humorous anecdotes identify him as an experienced clinician and add rhetorical power to his advice on how to talk with patients. By providing students with an alternative model of professional identity, Daniel's teaching could be seen as undermining customary practices. He advocates a way of relating to patients which can be characterised as dialogical or authentically patient-centred, because it respects patients' agency, emotions and individual history, and affirms their humanity. However, he fails to address the limits to students' agency, and the barriers to them seeking free and informed consent from patients in the presence of doctors. A student's subordinate position limits their influence over the way patients are approached, and he offers no advice as to how a student might respond if asked by a doctor to perform an examination when valid consent has not been obtained.

Students commonly witness and participate in consent practices that deviate from recommended protocols. These include withholding information about a students' status or presence, failing to give patients the option of having the procedure done by a more experienced person and the assumption that a patient's silence implies consent. These are represented in students' stories as customary practices rather than occasional lapses and are often defended on the grounds that they are necessary to enable students to gain sufficient access to patients. However, patients are not under a moral obligation to participate in student teaching, even though many doctors appear to hold this belief (Waterbury,

2001). Practices built on this assumption disregard patients' right to choose whether to accept the risk of additional discomfort involved in allowing an inexperienced person to carry out a procedure or examination.

Such practices shape the emerging professional identity of students, when they begin to identify patients as adversaries. They observe doctors using their position of power to exert pressure on patients, or to withhold information about students' presence. This way of relating to patients could affect students' future disclosure and consent practices once they are qualified. They might limit their disclosure of differential diagnoses and treatment choices, or their reasons for choosing a particular option. This is because, when seeking consent or choosing what information to disclose and how to go about it, they may not recognise the inevitable power imbalance. As a result, they may not be able to appreciate the fact that a patient could have difficulty expressing a view that differs from that of the doctor.

Clinical educators should pay attention to the unease some students experience in the face of customary practices, such as that described by Thao, and the ambivalence implied by Grace. Attributing such troubling feelings to personal weakness or a failure of socialisation into the profession is likely to dissuade students from expressing them. It would be better to acknowledge them as an indicator of conflict between customary practices and their established identities. This could draw attention to the need to consider and discuss whether some practices they are expected to follow are ethically problematic.

When it comes to obtaining consent to patients' involvement in students' clinical education, teaching students *how* to obtain valid consent is not sufficient to ensure that these practices will be followed. Students are heavily influenced by the practices and attitudes of those clinicians with whom they are seeking to identify, even though they sometimes perform acts of resistance. They often find themselves in situations where their own interests and those of their peers or clinical teachers appear to conflict with those of the patient. An adversarial attitude towards patients is associated with commonly accepted practices which deny patients their right to choose whether to participate in students' education. Power relationships and students' subordinate position in relation to doctors can render them unable to articulate their concerns when proper consent has not been obtained for examinations or procedures. This can echo the disempowerment that the patients themselves are likely to experience.

However, these stories also demonstrate that identity formation is not a passive process of enculturation. As demonstrated in this chapter, students actively resist some of the expectations placed upon them by cultural practices. Thao maintains his opposition to the surgeon's attitude even though he complies with the request to carry out the examination of a woman's breast. Grace declines to take blood without supervision or to attempt to do so when it has been unsuccessful at the first try, even when asked to do so. When they carry out these subtle acts of resistance, students emphasise their own agency (Rees & Monrouxe, 2011).

In the next chapter, I bring together three stories of one particular bedside teaching encounter, examining the different meanings generated from the event for the patient being examined, one of the students watching, and myself as participant-observer. The tutorial is revealed as a complex situation which can be a site for contention and a breeding ground for confusion. The analysis and discussion of these stories draws on the findings from previous chapters.

Note

* This chapter contains material adapted from a previously published article by Sally Warmington and Geoff McColl (2016): 'Medical student stories of participation in patient care-related activities: the construction of relational identity', in *Advances in Health Sciences Education*. Permission granted by Springer Nature for publication in this book.

References

Australian Medical Council. (2014). *Good medical practice – a code of conduct for doctors in Australia* (pp. 1–25). Medical Board of Australia. Retrieved from: www.medicalboard.gov.au/Codes-Guidelines-Policies/Code-of-conduct.aspx

Australian Medical Council Limited. (2010). Standards for the assessment and accreditation of medical schools by the Australian Medical Council 2010. Retrieved from www.amc.org.au/images/Medschool/accreditation-standards-medical-schools-2010.pdf

Coldicott, Y., Pope, C., & Roberts, C. (2003). The ethics of intimate examination. *British Medical Journal, 326*, 97–101.

DelVecchio Good, M.-J. (2011). The inner life of medicine: A commentary on anthropologies of clinical training in the twenty-first century. *Culture, Medicine and Psychiatry, 35*, 321–327. doi:10.1007/s11013-011-9217-z

Frank, A. W. (2002). 'How can they act like that?' Physicians and patients as characters in each other's stories. *Hastings Center Report, 32*(6), 14–22.

Frank, A. W. (2010). *Letting stories breathe: A socio-narratology.* Chicago, IL & London: University of Chicago Press.

Ginsburg, S., Regehr, G., & Lingard, L. (2003). The disavowed curriculum: Understanding students' reasoning in professionally challenging situations. *Journal of General Internal Medicine, 18*, 1015–1022.

Guillemin, M., & Gillam, L. (2006). *Telling moments: Everyday ethics in health care.* Melbourne: IP Communications.

Hartz, M. B., & Beal, J. R. (2000). Patients' attitudes and comfort levels regarding medical students' involvement in obstetrics-gynecology outpatient clinics. *Academic Medicine, 75*(10), 1010–1014.

Hendrickx, K., De Winter, B. Y., Wyndaele, J.-J., Tjalma, W. A. A., Debaene, L., Selleslags, B., … Bossaert, L. (2006). Intimate examination teaching with volunteers: Implementation and assessment at the University of Antwerp. *Patient Education and Counseling, 63*(1–2), 47–54.

Holmes, S., Jenks, A., & Stonington, S. (2011). Clinical subjectivation: Anthropologies of contemporary biomedical training. *Culture, Medicine and Psychiatry, 35*, 105–112. doi:10.1007/s11013-011-9207-1

Lemke, J. L. (2008). Identity, development and desire: Critical questions. In C. R. Caldas-Coulthard & R. Iedema (Eds.), *Identity trouble: Critical discourse and contested identities* (pp. 17–42). Basingstoke & New York: Palgrave Macmillan.

Medical Board of Australia. (2009). *Good medical practice: A code of conduct for doctors in Australia.* (p. 19).

Monrouxe, L. (2010). Identity, identification and medical education: Why should we care? *Medical Education, 44*(1), 40–49. doi:10.1111/j.1365-2923.2009.03440.x

Rees, C., Knight, L., & Wilkinson, C. (2007). Doctors being up there and we being down there: A metaphorical analysis of talk about student/doctor relationships. *Social Science and Medicine, 65,* 725–737.

Rees, C., & Monrouxe, L. V. (2008). 'Is it alright if I-um-we unbutton your pyjama top now?' Pronominal use in bedside teaching encounters. *Communication and Medicine, 5*(2), 171–182.

Rees, C., & Monrouxe, L. V. (2011). Medical students learning intimate examinations without valid consent: A multicentre study. *Medical Education, 45*(3), 261–272. doi:10.1111/j.1365-2923.2010.03911.x

Robertson, K., Hegarty, K., O'Connor, V., & Gunn, J. (2003). Women teaching women's health: Issues in the establishment of a clinical teaching associate program for the well woman check. *Women & Health, 37*(4), 49–65. doi:10.1300/J013v37n04_05

Roccas, S., Sagiv, L., Schwartz, S., Halevy, N., & Eidelson, R. (2008). Toward a unifying model of identification with groups: Integrating theoretical perspectives. *Personality and Social Psychology Review, 12*(3), 280–306. doi:10.1177/1088868308319225

Silver-Isenstadt, A., & Ubel, P. A. (1999). Erosion in medical students' attitudes about telling patients they are students. *Journal of General Internal Medicine, 14*(8), 481–487.

Taylor, J. S. (2011). The moral aesthetics of simulated suffering in standardized patient performances. *Culture, Medicine and Psychiatry, 35,* 134–162. doi:10.1007/s11013-011-9211-5

Waterbury, J. T. (2001). Refuting patients' obligations to clinical training: A critical analysis of the arguments for an obligation of patients to participate in the clinical education of medical students. *Medical Education, 35*(3), 286–294.

Wenger, E. (1998). *Communities of practice: Learning, meaning and identity.* Cambridge: Cambridge University Press.

World Medical Association. (2006 [1949]). *International Code of Medical Ethics.* (p. 2). Retrieved from: https:/wma.net/policies-post/wma-international-code-of-medical-ethics/

7 Complexity, contest and confusion

> So, what you learnt at uni [about communicating with patients], is that easy to put into practice here?
>
> It's hard to say. I mean, it does help, but there's a hundred other things that makes it even more complicated, you know? I mean, it's almost that – um – it gets to a stage where, towards the end, you're not even too worried about how you speak to the patient because – you've had that experience – you've got bigger fish to fry, you know? You make sure you get the techniques right; don't want to look like a fool in front of the examiner; things like that.
>
> Max, medical student

Perspectives on a bedside teaching encounter

In this passage, Max admits that when students are being assessed, demonstrating technical competence and avoiding the shame of failure seem more important to them than how they speak to a patient. 'You've got bigger fish to fry' because poor technical performance could affect your evaluation and, potentially, your future career. Through his use of the pronoun 'you' to refer to himself and his peers, Max limits his personal responsibility for prioritising his own interests (Rees & Monrouxe, 2008). Through his metaphor 'bigger fish to fry' he conveys the idea that something is at stake which is more important than the quality of his communication.

In this chapter, I explore the interactions taking place in a bedside tutorial through the eyes of three storytellers: myself, one of the students watching the examination, and the patient being examined. Through the juxtaposition of these stories, insights emerge into the diverse meanings of a bedside teaching encounter, the ways power is assumed and contested and its relationship with identity construction.

Researcher's story: narrative silencing

My story of the bedside teaching encounter has been reconstructed from field notes written during and immediately after the event. It is one of many possible interpretations of events, since stories are always structured and told from a particular perspective and designed for their intended audience. This potential limitation is offset by the inclusion and juxtaposition of audio-recorded data from interviews with two other participants in the encounter: Grace, one of the students watching, and Brian, the patient. The audio-recorded data allows access to the words and expressions used, as well as non-verbal material such as vocal volume, intonation and hesitations, and ambient environmental sounds. After presenting the main findings from the dialogic analysis of the three stories, I offer accounts of other ways clinical teachers can respond to unexpected disruptions during a tutorial and discuss the findings in relation to relevant literature.

The neurological examination

I arrive on the ward for the late afternoon tutorial and greet the waiting students. We talk about the fact that their end-of-year exams are only a few weeks away, which lends a sense of urgency to proceedings. I am looking forward to this session because, on the basis of my interview with Nick and observations of his teaching, I believe him to be a good teacher and caring doctor. During our interview, Nick said he didn't like to push reluctant students into doing physical examinations, but he knew this could disadvantage less confident students. His aim was for them to go beyond asking a routine list of questions, to listen to the patient's stories and pay attention to their concerns.

After he arrives, we follow Nick to a nearby ward and wait by the door of a shared room, while he approaches a white-haired man lying in bed wearing a dressing gown over a white hospital gown. Nick introduces himself and explains he is teaching some students. 'Would it be OK if one of them examines you?' he asks. The man agrees and Nick beckons us in from the corridor. Nick tells us that Mr Smith was admitted with arm weakness and asks Walid to carry out a neurological examination of his upper limbs, in less than eight minutes.

Walid is a quiet student, born and educated in a South-East Asian country, who came to Australia to study medicine. When I interviewed him earlier in the year, he told me that he wanted to 'console [patients] in times of illness and health'. He told me that communication with patients was difficult for him, despite having learnt English from an early age, because of the multitude of different accents and Australian colloquial expressions he encountered. He felt that his apprehension limited his ability to empathise with patients.

Walid approaches the bed and introduces himself:

'Hello, Mr Smith, my name is Walid'.

'Pleased to meet you – call me Brian'.

Both smile as they shake hands. We gather around the bed, Walid on Brian's right, and Nick at the foot of the bed. I am on the left with the other students and, like them, I have my notebook and pen in hand. I notice that there are no cards, flowers or personal belongings on Brian's bedside locker.

'Is it OK if I examine you?' asks Walid. 'I will look at your upper limbs and shoulders. We'll take off your robe if you don't mind'.

As Walid removes Brian's dressing gown with Nick's help, it is clear he has trouble moving his left arm. 'Thank you', he says, once Brian is settled back on the pillows.

'I had 55 years at Vic Rail. I used to go to a boxing class for five years. I went there after work every Tuesday and Thursday', offers Brian.

'OK. Excellent. Now let's go on with the examination', directs Nick. 'What about his general appearance?'

'He seems to have an IV cannula in his elbow and not much movement of his left hand'.

'What about the posture of his limbs – the position?'

'His left hand is clenched, and the elbow extended'.

Urging him to observe Brian more closely, Nick asks: 'What about his face?'

'He looks tired'.

Nick makes his question more specific. 'Is there any asymmetry of his face?'

Walid scrutinises Brian's face for a long time but says nothing. When Brian smiles at another student, his mouth droops on the left and Walid remarks on this asymmetry. Returning to Brian's arms, he reports there is wasting of the muscles of the left arm.

'I played lawn bowls for a few years, at Sunny Grove Country Club', says Brian. 'Good', says Nick. Then to Walid: 'Is the muscle wasting localised or generalised?' Walid decides it's generalised and then comments on the bruises on Brian's arms. 'They've been taking blood out of my arms for the last three days or so, for blood tests', Brian informs us. Nick responds: 'Yeah'.

Walid examines the muscle tone in Brian's arms. 'Relax your arm, make it floppy', he says. After moving Brian's arms to test the muscles' resistance to movement, he reports: 'There is increased tone in both, but especially on the left'. He examines the strength in Brian's arms, finding that his left hand is weaker, and for several minutes, Brian follows his instructions but does not speak. Then he remarks: 'Before I had the stroke, I used to be able to play the piano, but now I can't. It was the left hand that was affected with the piano'. Walid replies: 'You mentioned that the left hand was affected the most?' However, before Brian can respond, Nick interjects: 'Don't take a history; just examine'.

Walid continues examining Brian's arms and reporting his findings to Nick. He says he will look for neglect, a neurological deficit that makes it more difficult to notice things on the affected side of the body. 'I was diagnosed with left sided neglect', offers Brian. Nick interjects: 'Don't tell him, see if he can guess'. But Brian continues: 'Left sided neglect is when you're walking down a footpath and a shrub pokes out, and you virtually don't see it and walk into it'.

'Now, I'm going to test your reflexes', says Walid. Brian is unable to relax his arms, so Walid is unsuccessful at eliciting reflexes. Nick patiently shows him how to position the arm, place his own finger over the biceps tendon and strike it with the hammer. Walid is unable to elicit any jerks after two more attempts, even after Nick demonstrates, speaking loudly and clearly: 'Brian, I am going to ask you to fold your arms and I will tap gently'. So far, the examination has taken at least 15 minutes and is far from complete. At this point, Brian closes his eyes for a minute or two.

Walid asks Brian to perform a series of rapid alternating movements with his hands to assess his co-ordination. He is unable to do so and ends up with his hands in a prayer position. Smiling, he says: 'I'm going to say a prayer for you'.

'You've got to engage them', says Nick, then loudly and authoritatively, he says: 'Brian, look at me. Put your right hand on top of your left and do this'. He demonstrates the movements, but Brian's efforts to imitate him dissolve into clapping. Smiling again, he says 'I'm clapping their performance'. Walid attempts another test, trying to get Brian to move his finger back and forth between his nose and Walid's fingertip, but he can't do it and Nick again demonstrates the technique. 'It's dragging out a bit now', says Brian.

'We're nearly done – only another three minutes', answers Nick.

'It's becoming a drag', Brian says.

'Nearly done', repeats Nick. Walid starts to test sensation, which requires Brian to close his eyes; but Brian doesn't appear to detect the touch on his leg.

'Leave it', says Nick, 'He's having trouble understanding. See if he can co-operate with testing proprioception'.

'One last test'. Nick tells Brian and shows Walid the technique, but Brian can't follow his instructions and, afterwards, Walid has to ask three times before Brian opens his eyes.

'He's having trouble understanding. What else would you like to do?' says Nick.

Walid starts to examine Brian's legs but again has difficulty eliciting reflexes, and Nick demonstrates, saying: 'He might not co-operate'. He supports Brian's knees and tells him to relax, eliciting reflex jerks from his knees and ankles, which are more pronounced on the left. 'I'm going to tickle your feet for a sec', advises Nick. When he draws a line along the sole of Brian's right foot with his nail, Brian pulls away but his big toe flexes down. 'Sorry. A bit uncomfortable', he says to Brian. He repeats the test on the left and this time the toes flare outwards, and the big toe goes up. This is a positive Babinski sign, consistent with his stroke. To Brian he says again: 'Sorry'. Then to Walid and the group: 'Upgoing. Good'.

After more than half an hour, Nick decides it's time to finish so they thank Brian and move to another room to discuss the case. Before following them, I offer to help put Brian's dressing gown back on. 'It might be warmer', he says. As I help with the sleeves, I enquire: 'So you were a bowler and a boxer, were you?'

'Yes, an amateur boxer. It was a big part of my life back then'.

The effect of this brief exchange is dramatic. Brian's face, previously flat and expressionless, lights up with a smile. I tell him I am looking for people to interview for my research and ask if he would be willing, and he says he would be happy to talk to me the next day. 'My name's Sally', I say, and we shake hands. 'Thank you very much', he says as I adjust the bedclothes. Then with a mischievous smile, he remarks, 'That sounds like Elvis'. We both laugh and I depart saying: 'I'll see you tomorrow'.

Narrative silencing and the eloquent body

For me, the most striking feature of this interaction is the response to Brian's attempts to tell stories. Each time he begins, Nick shuts him down before continuing to direct the examination. This is an instance of narrative silencing, which indicates that Nick sees no place for Brian's stories in this context (Gubrium & Holstein, 2009, p. 52). Figure 7.1 illustrates how each of the story fragments offered by Brian are somehow related to what is going on in the tutorial. He offers the information about boxing after Nick and Walid talk about examining his arms, and about playing lawn bowls in response to Walid's scrutiny of his arms and the talk about muscle wasting. After weakness and loss of co-ordination in his left hand is noted, he tells how a previous stroke affected his ability to play the piano. When neglect is mentioned he offers a story about walking into a shrub. There is no response to indicate that anyone observed the connections between his stories and what was happening.

During the interaction, Nick and Walid engage in what has been described as *back-stage* talk: speaking rapidly and quietly to each other using medical jargon (Monrouxe, Rees, & Bradley, 2009). This is designed to exclude the patient, but Brian fails to play his expected role and responds to their conversation. His unorthodox participation can be understood variously as evidence of impaired cognitive function, a lack of awareness of the role in which he has been cast, or an act of resistance. Brian's story fragments are an example of intertextuality and a key focus of interest in my account. If Nick and the students fail to appreciate the connections between the examination and Brian's opening storylines,

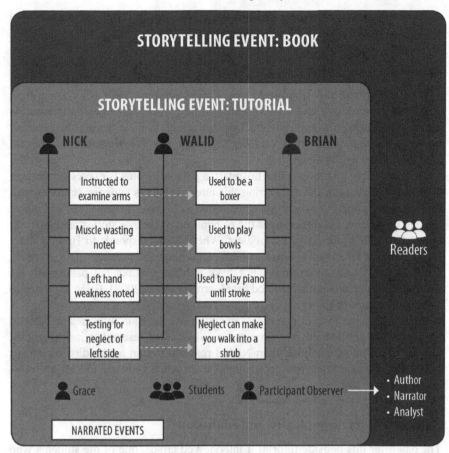

Figure 7.1 Tutorial with Brian, Walid and Nick.

his remarks might suggest that he is confused. When I interview Grace the following day, I discover that this was in fact her interpretation.

At the start of the tutorial, Brian tries to engage with the group by smiling and asking Walid to call him by his first name. After several of his story fragments are met with disinterest, he appears perplexed, then his face becomes expressionless and he seems to withdraw into himself. A similar change in another patient was described following objectifying treatment during a bedside teaching encounter: 'His mood changed dramatically from happy and joking at the start to looking blank, unsmiling and stunned soon after' (Monrouxe et al., 2009, p. 923). For a long period, Brian does not speak and after being told to close his eyes, it takes three requests for him to open them again. I wonder whether this is because he is tired, hard of hearing or trying to escape from the situation. His attempts to engage the group with his remarks about his hand movements also fail to elicit a response. Those comments might also have been an attempt to cover up his inability to perform the co-ordination tests. Brian's change in demeanour is rapidly reversed when I engage him in conversation after the group has left, acknowledging his stories.

Relationships and status

Several students in this group told me of their admiration for Nick, describing him as a caring doctor and a good teacher. They would have been motivated to please him during the tutorial and by succeeding in their exams. In contrast, their relationship with Brian was fleeting; they had not seen him before and probably never would again.

In hierarchical institutions like hospitals, a person's status is expressed through their interactions with others. During this tutorial, Nick's superior status in relation to students and the patient is demonstrated as he gives instructions, and others comply with them. He discourages the elaboration of Brian's stories, and instructs him not to tell Walid about his neglect. When Walid responds to Brian's statement about the effects of his stroke on his piano playing, Nick interrupts, advising him that he is only to examine, not 'take a history'. Like the patients in the bedside teaching encounters studied by Monrouxe et al. (2009), Brian is related to at different stages of the event as an *active participant* and as a *non-person*.

Nick's decision to continue the examination when Brian indicates he has had enough is not challenged. My own status as a student researcher is ambiguous; although I am more qualified than Nick, I respond to him as the director of this performance and refrain from interrupting, even when I can see that Brian wants it to finish.

Student's story: complexity and confusion

The day after this bedside tutorial, I interviewed Grace, one of the students who observed events unfold. An Australian-born woman of South-East Asian heritage, Grace was quietly spoken and thoughtful. She told me that her volunteer work at a soup kitchen for homeless people had increased her capacity to interact with patients confidently and empathise with those whose backgrounds differed from her own. We talked about why hospital patients might agree to be involved in students' education. She said that, since they have little to do, there is no reason for them to refuse. She also remarked that because students wear stethoscopes around their necks, they might be mistaken for doctors.

Grace admitted that it could be difficult for a patient to say no, even if they would rather not participate. Her usual approach was to say: 'I'm a medical student. Is it OK if I chat with you for a bit?' Most patients agreed to be seen when she put the request in these terms. She would not usually say that seeing them was optional, but if they looked reluctant, she would offer to come back later. Grace said that students only get to see patients in pain or distress when they are with a doctor, and that patients rarely refuse a doctor's request. Even patients who were hesitant at the start of a teaching session would usually relax as it went on, leading her to conclude that their apprehension was related to a fear of the unknown. I asked how she thought Brian had felt about being seen by the students the previous day.

I wasn't too sure, myself. I think he was OK with it, it seemed and – [pause] sorry, he seemed – um – um [pause]. I'm not too sure the basis of his confusion, whether he was like that all the time, or maybe he was just confused in that setting, or um …

So, what made you feel he was confused?

Um – [pause] I think, um, oh … just responding to the questions that – um – the other student posed and um … I think, after a while, he looked around at us a lot for a bit, and I think, after a while he sort of lost interest and asked, you know, when this would finish and um – [pause] you know?

So, he wanted it to end?

Yeah. Well, I think, um – [pause] I think, in that particular patient, um – he wasn't too sure as to what was happening, and I think in tutorials, this happens more than other times, when there's a student doctor and an actual doctor there. And the interaction between the two, and sort of the purpose as to why they're examining the patient, and I think it's confusing to them because sometimes it can drag on for a long time and they seem to repeat a lot of things and there's a lot of sort of looking, and things aren't as succinct as what a student would do by themselves, and what a doctor would do for the management of the patient.

Do you mean that the patient isn't clear about what's supposed to be happening?

Yeah, because I think there's also some confusion in the student as well, who examines the patient. And when you have someone else who's examining you but sort of in a tentative way, then I think the patient isn't sure about what's happening either and whether he should be looking at the student or the doctor, and like if there's a crowd as well. So – um – ah – um – in the patient yesterday, I think he seemed quite comfortable with it. Um – [pause] yeah. He just seemed to have some trouble – um – understanding the directions for the examination, and I think maybe just got confused in that aspect for a while. As in: 'I'm not too sure what they want me to do and why everyone else has to watch this – this happening'.

Yeah, sure. OK. So it's quite a complicated situation … to have the student and the tutor and the people watching?

I think so, yeah. And you know, it wasn't just that student. I think a lot of students become – a bit apprehensive in a tutorial setting. Yeah, and – sometimes we – we – can forget about the patient that's there, because we're concentrating too much on our technique or what's going to come next, and looking right for the doctor. … So, when you're a student by yourself, you focus on the patient – [pause] 90 per cent and you can tell if they're uncomfortable, and halfway through you ask them if they're all right, if we can keep going, and so on. In a tutorial you're doing a lot of other things, sort of, at the same time. You're aware of all these people watching you. You're reporting back to the tutor. You're trying to take on what – the advice of the tutor, and watch what he does, and repeat it, and then move on and have your differentials list in your mind. Even though we're supposed to be doing this by ourselves as well, it's – um – it is a bit more pressure. ... So we don't tend to focus on, sort of, the comfort of the patient so much, I think in a tutorial setting.

Not as much as you would as an individual?

Mmm, because you would notice it more, I think. And so that might add to the patient's apprehension, and so on.

Yeah, OK. It's very interesting, that whole setting of the tutorial, because there's so much going on.

Yeah. I have never actually thought about it. So, sorry it took so long to get out, but –

No problem, because it is something you need to stop and think about.

Complexity generates confusion

Grace responds to my question about how she thinks Brian was feeling, saying she thought he was OK with it, but that he seemed confused. She suggests possible reasons for his apparent confusion, including the interaction between student and tutor, the uncertainty about the reason for the examination, its tentative and repetitive nature and Brian's difficulty understanding the directions. She describes Walid's apprehension as a common experience, made worse by the competing demands of the situation. Grace says these factors limit students' capacity to focus on patients' needs, which they do better when seeing them alone.

I consider the analysis of this excerpt in two parts. In the first part, Grace's performance is hesitant, full of pauses, filler words and repetitions; she precedes her remarks 12 times with the phrase 'I think'. This functions as a hedge, mitigating the potential for a negative response from her audience by suggesting that Grace is uncertain of her position (Rees & Monrouxe, 2008). There is a tension between her statement – 'I think he seemed quite comfortable with it' and her observation that Brian was confused about what was going on, had lost interest and wanted the examination to finish. She tries to imagine what the experience might have been like for Brian and why it might have been confusing.

In the second part, Grace speaks more confidently, drawing on her own experience as she describes how a student's solo encounter with a patient differs from their involvement in a tutorial. She uses the expression 'I think' only three times in the second part of the passage. She repeatedly employs the plural pronoun 'you', which has the rhetorical effect of persuading the audience to accept a statement as 'a generally admitted "truth"' (Rees & Monrouxe, 2008, p. 172). She uses it to evoke a students' experience in a tutorial situation, listing the tasks simultaneously facing them as they try to deal with the demands of the situation. She also employs the pronoun 'we' to refer to herself and her peers when she says: 'We forget about the patient' and 'We don't tend to focus on the comfort of the patient so much'. This has the effect of abrogating responsibility from the speaker (Rees & Monrouxe, 2008, p. 172).

The pronoun 'we' here might be interpreted as including the tutor, except that soon afterwards, she says 'and looking right for the doctor'. This suggests that it refers to the students, implying that it is their responsibility to take care of the patient. Grace is silent about the tutor's position of authority, and the power dynamics which virtually preclude students from expressing concern about a patient's discomfort, especially if the tutor may have contributed to it. Grace's positive regard for this tutor could be another obstacle to her implying any criticism of Nick for the inattention of the group to Brian's needs. She does not draw a link between Brian's lack of understanding of what is required of him and the cursory way Nick requested his participation.

Dual 'voices' and an evolving identity

This story can be understood as a multi-vocal narrative, similar to those of Daniel and Ashanka in earlier chapters. Between the first and second parts of this passage, Grace is hesitant, as if reluctant to express a definite opinion without hedging; this may be related to the fact that she is working hard to imagine and empathise with the experience of the patient. Another possible explanation is that she is experiencing identity dissonance brought about by the conflict between her established identities valuing altruism and integrity, and the practices and values expected of her emerging professional identity. She is hesitant and uncertain, embodying the confusion she describes in the patient and the student examining him.

In the second part, her voice is more assured as she describes the experience of a student carrying out an examination during a tutorial. This is familiar territory, since she has first-hand experience of the situation. She constructs a coherent story in which complexity and competing demands explain the relative inattention to the patient's needs. She acknowledges the undesirable effects on the patient, accepting some responsibility for the situation. By constructing this explanation, she identifies herself as a person with agency, and acknowledges the existence of a problem. However, she does not acknowledge the tutor's responsibility for the way events unfolded.

Grace apologises for taking so long to articulate her thoughts and explains that she has never considered these matters before. This confirms once again how research interviews can be a site for the dialogical construction of identity through storytelling (Tanggaard, 2009). It also suggests that, even though Grace has been taught that the patient's perspective is important, it has not been explored in relation to the tutorial context.

Patient's story: a boring operation

The morning after the tutorial, I arrived at Brian's bedside to find him wearing a white hospital gown under his dressing gown, as he had the evening before. The interview took place in a shared ward, with the usual distractions: staff going in and out to speak with patients or respond to incessantly beeping equipment.

While I spoke with Brian, I had the impression that his thinking was slowed, and it was difficult to get him to follow a change in topic. Sometimes, when I thought we had finished talking about one topic and asked him about something else, he would have something more to say about the first topic before being ready to move on. This might also have been because we had different priorities and expectations of the conversation. After I had gathered plenty of stories about his interactions with students, I followed the conversation wherever Brian led me, and a wealth of information about his life emerged. His stories allowed me to place some of his earlier remarks in context and accomplished substantial identity work. I discovered he had been a railway employee, had run a milk bar with his wife and had been a keen amateur performer in a light opera company.

The following excerpt begins when I ask Brian about the previous day's tutorial.

What was it like for you when they were there, and one of them was examining you?

I got tired of that – of that session.

Yeah, I thought you did. So, it went on for a long time?

Oh – it's all dragged out. And the bloke that he had – conducting a session on me – he wasn't very good, was he? Well, I mean, you couldn't understand what he was talking about half the time. For what he did, you could have cut it down in time – down to about five minutes.

Yeah, right. So, when the doctor came to ask you … did you think it was going to be a lot shorter?

Nowhere near as long as it did take.

And I guess the other thing is that um – you didn't get a chance to have much of a talk with them, did you?

I didn't think, the chap that he got to do the – the testing on me; he didn't seem to impart what he was doing to the rest of the people … while he was doing it, he was supposed to be explaining things to them, at the same time. None of that was going over to anybody at all really. … At one stage I said to the main bloke that was here with the student with him – I said – I said it's dragging out a bit. I said it's a real drag. It was a real drag.

Yeah, and how did he respond to that?

[Pause] He – he got the idea that I wanted to – sort of fizzle down to – to a finito.

Did it finish quick enough, or did it still drag on after that?

It didn't finish anywhere near as – quick as it should have been.

So, it still dragged on a bit after that, you thought?

Yeah, it did – it got too <u>boring</u>. Was a <u>boring</u> operation.

Were you hoping that seeing them would involve a bit more of a chat, like, you'd like to be able to tell them something? Or that they would be interested to hear your story?

There was nothing I could think of that would have been any good. [Sounds wistful]

Well – I noticed that you tried to tell them a few things; but they were focused on the examination, I think.

Yeah, they were definitely – [long pause] linked right in. Right into the – examination side of it.

Did you feel like they were seeing you as a person or was it more that they were seeing you as someone to practice on?

Yeah, I was just a practice, piece of <u>machinery.</u> Practising on a – on a car that – hadn't been driven before. Yeah, that's what – about what it was.

So, you didn't like that? Is that what you're saying?

The hammer didn't – nothing responded to the hammer much at all really, but they got some satisfaction from it.

Yeah. Um – do you feel now that letting the students see you was – a helpful thing for them? Do you think they would have learnt something?

Well, they must have picked something up. They only just need one little thing to pick up, and restore that in their minds. ... I think after that whole session, they went off somewhere to group and talk together, between them, so that's where they would've got it probably.

Identity shifts

In response to my question as to what it was like for him during the examination, Brian says he got tired of it, it took longer than expected and continued after he told the tutor he wanted it to stop. He criticises Walid's performance, saying that he could not understand what Walid was saying, he did not convey his findings to the group, and he took too long. He seems to understand something of what is expected of students in a tutorial, despite Grace's impression that he was confused.

When I ask whether the students saw him as a person or something to practise on, he says that he had felt treated like a piece of machinery. He explains that he didn't give much thought to his decision to be involved in the tutorial, and that despite his boredom he hopes his participation was useful. Apart from his references to being bored, he seems more interested in criticising Walid's performance and discussing the potential for the students to benefit than describing his own feelings. In relation to the question as to whether he had hoped to have a chance to tell his story, he replies wistfully: 'There was nothing I could think of that would have been any good'.

Brian acknowledges that Nick was in charge of the tutorial and believes he knew Brian wanted it to finish. Despite being treated like a passive object for much of the time, he resists this when he attempts to tell stories about his life. In the interview context, Brian identifies himself as an easy-going, agreeable man who readily agreed to help the students. During the tutorial his identity shifts a number of times. At the outset, he appears alert, smiling and engaged with the audience but soon afterwards, he appears silent and withdrawn, adopting a blank facial expression or closing his eyes. Later he tries to engage them with his remarks about praying and clapping. These changes in his demeanour can be linked with shifts in his subject position from active to passive and back again, associated with the shifting stance taken towards him by Nick and Walid as an active participant and a non-person.

Responding creatively to disruption

During my fieldwork, I became aware of some tutors who acknowledged and responded to a patient's needs, even when they diverted attention from the task at hand. During a tutorial I attended led by Veronica, I was struck by the way she reacted when a patient being examined raised an issue of concern to her.

> The patient had recently suffered a stroke, causing paralysis of the left side of her body. As one of the students examined her abdomen, the patient suddenly declared: 'I'm a different Annie now'.

> 'You're different because your arm doesn't move the way it used to. But you are the same Annie up here'. Veronica pointed to her own head. 'I know, because I've seen your scans and I know what happened'.

> 'Do you really think so?'

> 'Yes, I do'. Veronica replied.

I raised this incident when I interviewed Veronica two weeks later.

> I remember now, I had to step in and acknowledge that for that patient, um – 'cos that was obviously a big thing for that patient, that – this is a crisis that she's going through that she thinks her life is just totally different now. I think I said to her, 'No, you're the same Annie in here, even though your body's different'.

Veronica's assertion that Annie was not changed as a person could be criticised for failing to validate her experience of her situation, and for trying to resolve such an existential question by reference to a scan. Nevertheless, I saw Veronica's response as a genuine attempt to acknowledge the patient's concerns. It contrasts with Nick's treatment of Brian, because she recognised that by responding sensitively, she was showing students that patients are not merely passive objects for teaching.

When I interviewed William, another tutor, he told me that empathy was an essential skill for students to learn.

> Personally, I think it's one of the most important things. Ah – however, I must say that because it's not taught of the tutors, ah – students gain that skill variably. Um – so, it's uneven across the board, even, you know, in this clinical school. Some tutors are well equipped to deal with the emotions of it, and some are not – ah – haven't developed it themselves, so cannot transmit it to the students. ... There's – there have been times in a tute where we were happily discussing something with a patient, and something triggers – so that the patient is crying in front of the tute. I break tute to counsel the patient and, you know, console and so forth – and the students actually find that the most interesting part of that tute [laughs] – because they've never been taught how to do that.

I asked him if he could tell me about any specific incidents he could remember.

> I had a patient [who] had a stroke, and – er – you know – it was – started off as a normal neurology examination of a stroke patient, eliciting the signs and so forth. And – er – one of the areas was speech, and there was a deficit in the stroke patient's speech. And the frustration in the inability to express themselves and so forth then broke down the patient. Um – and so, the students went 'Oh, what do we do here?' [Laughs] ... Like I say, it is actually only through those moments that you can actually walk your students through it. 'Cause if you talk it through a dry tute, it's organised learning rather than applicable learning. And that's what the clinical bedside tute offers, I think.

According to William, students find it particularly challenging to apply the knowledge acquired in their pre-clinical studies to a clinical context with patients who became distressed. He is always alert for the possibility of such pivotal moments arising during bedside teaching, because he believes that students can only develop the capacity to respond sensitively in future through witnessing and discussing real-life incidents like this. He reminds his students that:

> They should never forget that it is a privilege to treat a patient. A patient comes to you in their darkest hour and reaching out for need; and it is a privileged moment.

Veronica and William's stories show that for some tutors, disruptions of the intended learning activity by a patient can be tolerated, and even welcomed. They can be seen as valuable opportunities for students to learn how their interactions with a patient can provoke strong emotions, and how to respond to them sensitively.

Different stories, common threads

The analysis of material from multiple sources highlights the different meanings constructed by individuals witnessing the same events. As I observed the tutorial, I was struck by the rejection of Brian's attempts to tell his stories and by what I saw as his embodied expression of dejection and withdrawal in response. Grace's account focused on what she interpreted as confusion, most notably on the part of Brian, but also for Walid. She used the idea of confusion to explain their apparent uncertainty about what was expected of them. Brian drew attention to the protracted and boring nature of the interaction and the perceived shortcomings of Walid's performance, but felt his participation had been valuable.

Given his repeated attempts to interact with the students, it seems likely that Brian expected the tutorial to involve some kind of dialogue. He may have had conversations with students outside of a tutorial, when they had time to sit and listen. He does not realise that Nick expects him to behave in a passive way for much of the tutorial. Brian's actions might be seen by the tutor or students as transgressive, because he does not behave like a simulated patient, who would typically keep quiet unless addressed. In the absence of a debriefing to explore Brian's experience, there was no opportunity to mitigate any negative consequences.

Despite these differences, there is a common thread between these stories, which relates to shifting subject positions. As I observe the tutorial and recount my story, I shift between evaluating Brian's neurological deficits and Walid's performance and imagining Brian's experience. In Grace's story, she shifts from a hesitant voice when imagining the experience of a patient to a more confident one when she talks about a student's experience. Brian shifts between passively agreeing to the interaction and actively resisting the role in which he has been cast; between actively engaging with the audience and withdrawing into himself.

Recognising that clinical teaching interactions serve multiple purposes, Veronica and William acknowledge that disruptions to the expected course of a tutorial can be fruitful for students and patients, when managed sensitively. They also identify patients as both material for teaching and individuals whose stories are worthy of respect. These shifts in the observer's position with respect to those with whom they are interacting are analogous to the movements described earlier in relation to clinical interactions (Davenport, 2000; Katz & Shotter, 1996) or the dissection of cadavers in the anatomy laboratory (Hafferty, 1991).

Monrouxe et al. (2009) reflect on the work of Auge, incorporating the idea of *non-places*: temporary places of residence which have no particular associations for the person inhabiting them. Some patients can feel their sense of identity and self-worth is diminished by chronic illness even before they find themselves in hospital. In Brian's case there were no signs of any personal items in his vicinity that might have helped connect him to his identity – for example, there were no cards or flowers and no personal items apart from his dressing gown. The experience of being situated in a non-place and treated as a non-person – as in some clinical teaching situations – can lead to a sense of 'identity loss, low self-esteem, anonymity, and solitude' (Monrouxe et al., 2009, p. 928). Brian's expression of dejection and bewilderment and his sense of being treated like 'a piece of machinery' suggest that in this encounter, he may have experienced such a reaction.

Power dynamics and identity

Nick identifies himself as the person in charge of proceedings when he asks Brian to be involved. He is polite, but vague about what will be expected of Brian. Studies into patients' experiences of clinical teaching (Chretien, Goldman, Craven, & Faselis, 2010; Nair, Coughlan, & Hensley, 1997; Romano, 1941) recommend preparing patients before teaching events and offering them time to de-brief afterwards. During the introductions, Nick and Walid relate to Brian as a person, but once the 'serious business of teaching' begins, Brian is mostly identified as a prop or non-person (Monrouxe et al., 2009, p. 923).

Brian's opening storylines about his life can be interpreted as efforts to resist the denial of his identity. After his fourth attempt, about how an earlier stroke had affected his ability to play the piano, Walid acknowledges his remark, providing an opportunity for Brian to expand on his story, and for Walid to perform the empathic identity he is eager to develop. However, he is reprimanded by Nick and the story is shut down. This reinforces the fact that the recognition or denial of Brian's status as a person is mainly under Nick's control.

When Brian offers information about neglect, Nick instructs him not to say more, so that Walid can discover it from the examination. Through this exchange, Nick attempts to collude with Brian against Walid, and to do so, he has to relate to him as a person. In this case Brian does not go along with Nick's request, possibly because of hearing loss or cognitive impairment. His description about his experience of neglect, after he was asked not to tell Walid, could also be seen as an act of resistance. Towards the end of the examination, Nick briefly acknowledges Brian as a person when he apologises for the discomfort caused by testing his plantar reflexes, and again when he is thanked for his participation.

Nick requests Brian's participation with the assurance that comes with his position, knowing that patients are unlikely to refuse a doctor's request. Several times during the examination, he speaks to or about Brian in ways that could be considered demeaning, referring to him in his presence using third-person pronouns. When Walid's instructions don't seem to be getting through, he says to Walid: 'You have to engage them', and later: 'He's having trouble understanding' and 'He might not co-operate'.

Nick directs Walid to continue the examination, despite Brian's change in demeanour and his statement that it was 'a drag'. Despite his assurance that it will be only another few minutes, it continues for much longer, and I interpret this as another expression of Nick's powerful position. People may be unaware of the roles they perform in particular interactions and, given my impression of Nick's character, I believe he would have been unaware that he was relating to Brian as a passive object or non-person for much of the tutorial (Monrouxe et al., 2009).

The exercise of power is intimately related to the construction of identity. Nick identifies himself as a person of authority who expects to be obeyed, and as someone entitled to authorise or shut down other people's stories. In doing so, he limits Brian's capacity to construct an identity. Brian's embodied response is eloquent: his disengagement and loss of facial expression are striking, and so is his re-animation when I respond, albeit belatedly, to his stories. It is as though he responds to being treated as a non-person by temporarily becoming one. Walid struggles to construct an identity for himself in relation to Brian. His motivation to treat him with respect requires him to pay attention to Brian's story. Nick's rebuke when he shows interest in it disrupts Walid's identity performance as someone who respects Brian as a person.

Primacy of the student-doctor relationship

The findings of this chapter support the argument that treating patients as passive objects for teaching is a manifestation of the higher status of the student-doctor relationship in comparison with that between student and patient (Bleakley & Bligh, 2008). This tutorial offers a graphic illustration of Max's expression: 'You've got bigger fish to fry' – more important things to focus on – than the way you relate to a patient. Grace confirms this when she says that concentrating on technique and the tutor's appraisal can sometimes lead them to 'forget about the patient that's there'.

With Bleakley and Bligh (2008), I advocate an authentically patient-centred approach to clinical teaching and learning, enhancing the importance of the student-patient relationship. Following such a model, learning from patients with doctors as expert advisers would play an increasing role in many contexts. This would have an impact on the identities students construct in relation to patients. Diminishing the importance of role modelling and imitation, an appreciation of the differences between patients' experiences and their own would become more influential (Bleakley & Bligh, 2008; Bleakley, Bligh, & Browne, 2011).

Many of the ideas developed in earlier chapters are brought together through the analysis of these three stories about a particular bedside teaching encounter. The unacknowledged relational work of the interaction contributes to the construction and performance of identity for all those involved. It is intimately related to the dynamics of power and associated acts of resistance, as participants experience shifting subject positions and respond to complex and often competing demands. The priority given to the student-doctor relationship may contribute to the neglect of patients' needs in some clinical teaching events.

This chapter also explores the perceived tension between the interests of students and patients. For students there is much at stake, because they need to achieve technical mastery, and know that poor performance could derail their career plans. They also fear being exposed as incompetent in front of their teachers and peers. Clinical teachers want to help students succeed in their examinations, and may also be concerned about negative assessments of their teaching, if their students fail. For many patients, an opportunity to enter into a dialogue, to share with students something about their life or their illness experience is important. This need may not be articulated but it can be inferred from the stories they tell or, as in Brian's case, from their embodied response when their voices are silenced.

There is an apparent contradiction in the observation that a clinical teacher and a student who share a desire to treat patients humanely can engage in practices which treat a patient like a non-person. To understand this paradox, it is helpful to consider the context in which the encounter takes place, including the physical environment, and the time in relation to the impending examinations. The social and cultural context includes the relationships between the people involved in the interaction, as well as differences in status (Gubrium & Holstein, 2009). Teaching hospitals are deeply hierarchical, and this contributes to the ways in which power is exercised, and the difficulties in negotiating or contesting power for those in subordinate positions, such as students and patients.

Customary practices employed in clinical teaching are manifestations of the embedded cultural values of the profession. Although there are inevitably power disparities between teacher, student and patient, the exercise of power is rarely discussed in this context. As a result, opportunities are missed to consider the potential for misuse of that power (Rees, Ajjawi, & Monrouxe, 2013). The consent practices described in the previous chapter and further explored here may be used as a deliberate strategy to increase participation but could also result from unreflective compliance with customary practice.

The title of this chapter frames bedside teaching encounters as complex interactions, in which there can be a contest for power and identity, and in which many factors converge to produce a sense of confusion and misunderstanding. In the final chapter, I draw together threads from the previous chapters to make a case in favour of a dialogic medical education. The components of the final chapter encompass the contributions of this project to theory and methodology in relation to identity construction as well as opportunities for change on several levels. I consider the clinical encounter itself, curriculum design and delivery and wider institutional and professional contexts, proposing practical steps towards a dialogic medical education.

References

Bleakley, A., & Bligh, J. (2008). Students learning from patients: Let's get real in medical education. *Advances in Health Sciences Education, 13*, 89–107.

Bleakley, A., Bligh, J., & Browne, J. (2011). *Medical education for the future: Identity, power and location*. London: Springer.

Chretien, K., Goldman, E., Craven, K., & Faselis, C. (2010). A qualitative study of the meaning of physical examination teaching for patients. *Journal of General Internal Medicine, 25*(8), 786–791.

Davenport, B. A. (2000). Witnessing and the medical gaze: How medical students learn to see at a free clinic for the homeless. *Medical Anthropology Quarterly, 14*(3), 310–327.

Gubrium, J. F., & Holstein, J. A. (2009). *Analyzing narrative reality*. Los Angeles, CA: Sage.

Hafferty, F. W. (1991). *Into the valley: Death and the socialization of medical students*. New Haven, CT & London: Yale University Press.

Katz, A. M., & Shotter, J. (1996). Hearing the patient's 'voice': Toward a social poetics in diagnostic interviews. *Social Science and Medicine, 43*(6), 919–931.

Monrouxe, L., Rees, C., & Bradley, P. (2009). The construction of patients' involvement in hospital bedside teaching encounters. *Qualitative Health Research, 19*(7), 918–930. doi:10.1177/1049732309338583

Nair, B. R., Coughlan, J. L., & Hensley, M. J. (1997). Student and patient perspectives on bedside teaching. *Medical Education, 31*, 341–346.

Rees, C., Ajjawi, R., & Monrouxe, L. V. (2013). The construction of power in family medicine bedside teaching: A video observation study. *Medical Education, 47*(2), 154–165. doi:10.1111/medu.12055

Rees, C., & Monrouxe, L. V. (2008). 'Is it alright if I-um-we unbutton your pyjama top now?' Pronominal use in bedside teaching encounters. *Communication and Medicine, 5*(2), 171–182.

Romano, J. (1941). Patients' attitudes and behavior in ward round teaching. *JAMA (Chicago, Ill.), 117*(9), 664–667.

Tanggaard, L. (2009). The research interview as a dialogical context for the production of social life and personal narratives. *Qualitative Inquiry, 15*(9), 1498–1515.

8 Towards a dialogic medical education

> There is neither a first word nor a last word and there are no limits to the dialogic context; it extends into the boundless past and boundless future. Even past meanings, that is those born in the dialogue of past centuries, can never be stable – finalized, ended once and for all – they will always change – be renewed – in the process of subsequent, future development of the dialogue.
>
> (Bakhtin, 1986, p. 170)

To introduce this final chapter, I return to my aims in writing the book, which I outlined at the beginning, and look back on what has emerged from the intervening chapters. Bakhtin draws attention in the extract above to the fact that all communication is a link in an endless chain, responding to the words of others and anticipating a reply. Although these are the closing words of my dialogue with you, the reader, I make no claim to have uttered the last word on the subject. Like all spoken or written communication, this book responds to the words of others and calls for an answer in return. It is my response to the words written by other researchers and spoken during my fieldwork encounters and my experiences as a doctor and a patient. In turn, it calls for a reaction from the reader: perhaps a greater appreciation of the importance of storytelling, changes in practice or ideas for future research.

The dialogic analysis of stories gathered during this ethnographic project has enabled a deeper understanding of how identity is constructed relationally, and the kinds of identities that emerge in particular medical education contexts. Identities are constructed both <u>during</u> clinical encounters and when people talk <u>about</u> them, for example in conversations with their teachers and peers or in research interviews. In this chapter, I also explore the power dynamics of clinical teaching encounters that are revealed in some of the stories, along with ethically troubling practices that persist, even in medical schools which profess an ethos of patient-centredness.

Contexts of relational identity construction

Constructing identity in research interviews

When clinical teacher Daniel tells about the importance of storytelling in his everyday practice, he uses multiple voices to depict himself and other story characters in particular ways. By positioning himself in relation to them, he constructs an identity as a compassionate doctor. Similarly, student Ashanka tells about an interaction with her tutor using several voices to represent him and versions of herself. She juxtaposes these voices to construct an integrated identity for herself as a person who respects patient stories and to identify the tutor as someone who dismisses them.

These stories illustrate what I mean by the relational construction of identity and show how storytellers employ a variety of narrative devices to do this work. Bakhtin used the term *heteroglossia* to describe the fact that when using any language, narrators have available to them a multitude of different *speech genres* or voices (Bakhtin, 1981, 1986; Holquist, 2002). Each voice can indicate one or more of the social groups to which a speaker belongs, for example their nationality, age group, social class or occupation. In *multi-vocal* stories, like those told by Daniel and Ashanka, each voice conveys something about the narrator or one of their story characters.

Both these storytellers also use the narrative device of ventriloquation, speaking through the words of their story characters (Vågan, 2011). This means that, although the words of the staff in Daniel's story and those of Ashanka's tutor are presented as though they are direct quotes, those words have been chosen and performed by each narrator so as to represent those characters in a certain way. As narrators juxtapose their own voices with those of the other characters, they identify themselves as a particular kind of person in relation to them. This is the narrative device of interactional positioning (Wortham, 2000).

Constructing identity in clinical teaching encounters

In a medical tutorial, a patient named Mr Hartmann is interviewed by Anna, one of the students. Through the stories told during this interaction, he constructs a complex identity for himself as a self-reliant, resilient, well-informed, playful, humorous and driven individualist who does not reveal any concerns but is grateful for the care he has received. Anna skilfully makes space for his self-identifying stories while gathering disease-related information to present to her tutor, Robert. As a result, the tutorial becomes an occasion for Mr Hartmann's relational identity construction as parallel narratives of disease, illness experience and identity emerge. However, despite asserting his individuality, the stories that identify him as a particular kind of person are omitted from Anna's presentation of his case and Robert categorises him as a 'stock-standard patient'. As a result of the exclusion of personal stories from case presentations, students may learn to ignore characteristics of individual patients that could be relevant to their care.

During another tutorial, a patient named Brian also tries to tell autobiographical stories in response to what is happening, but in this case his stories are repeatedly shut down. There is very little opportunity for him to construct his identity, partly because he is involved in an examination, whereas Mr Hartmann and Anna were engaged in a history-taking exercise. However, if the tutor, Nick, had recognised what was going on and appreciated the importance of patients' stories, he could have made space for Brian to share something about himself before the examination. The narrative suppression Brian experienced during the tutorial appeared to have a profound effect on him, demonstrated by his disengagement from the group.

Illuminating patient experiences

When students talk about listening to patients' stories, they often imply this is something they will no longer have time for when they are qualified as doctors. They characterise it as a luxury that will need to be sacrificed for efficient medical practice. However, several of the stories in this book offer fresh insights into why these stories are told in this context and why they matter. We gain a rare understanding of some of the diverse experiences of patients when they participate in clinical teaching activities. The relationship between identity construction and power dynamics is also revealed, and ethical issues are raised that are rarely articulated or addressed in the context of clinical teaching.

Imagining the students' world

A patient named Peter offers a surprising view of his interactions with students, using interactional positioning to characterise them as child-like and himself as a parental figure. He represents them as timid, embarrassed and clumsy, and in need of his help; he is willing to let them examine him or carry out a procedure, despite having to endure extra discomfort. Peter demonstrates empathy for students, as he imagines their emotional state and is moved to alleviate their discomfort. During his hospitalisation, Peter has had to cope with numerous investigations, some of which were carried out without warning or explanation, and which left him feeling vulnerable and powerless. His encounters with students offer him an opportunity to construct an identity as a helpful and confident person in relation to them, which gives him a sense of empowerment. This points to a potential benefit from his participation, as he depicts himself as having chosen to be involved in their learning.

Harvey's story about an interaction with students also enables him to construct an identity as a stoic and confident man, an old hand in the hospital after multiple admissions who wants to help the students. However, unlike Peter, he forms a negative opinion about one student's character, deciding that he is arrogant. Harvey feels that this student wants to take something from him, as opposed to him giving it freely. His interpretation of the student's motivation may have led him to see his actions as a threat to his construction of an identity as a generous person, intensifying his antagonism. As a result, he withdraws his co-operation from that student and offers another one the opportunity to examine him.

During our research interview, Harvey's story about an 'arrogant' student was preceded by an account of a past episode of serious respiratory illness, which

required his admission to intensive care. When listening to the interview recording afterwards, I discovered to my regret that I had interrupted that story to question him about his interactions with students. After the 'arrogant student' story
he told me one about an 'arrogant doctor' he had encountered in his teens. The
sequence of stories, illustrated in Figure 4.2, can be interpreted as performing
identity work in relation to myself as his interviewer, suggesting that he may
have perceived me as arrogant as well, because I interrupted his first story to
focus on my own interests. This is one instance in which the multi-layered nature
of the storytelling events comes into sharp focus. The analysis encompasses not
only the identity construction taking place in relation to the narrated events, but
also in the storytelling event of the research interview. The Bakhtinian concept
of *emergence* is relevant here – it refers to the fact that the context in which a
story is told contributes to its meaning, as well as the story itself.

Object or active participant

Robin is frustrated by the fact that several days after his admission to hospital,
he has not had the opportunity for a meaningful conversation with his hospital
doctor. This problem is unexpectedly resolved in a blurring of boundaries
between our research interview and a clinical encounter with his doctor. When
his doctor arrives during a break in our interview, the chair which I had placed
beside Robin's bed prompted the doctor to sit down for the first time, helping
Robin to ask a vital question about his illness. Robin describes how he has been
engaged in teaching as an active participant, which he finds much more satisfying than the more common experience of being used by students as a 'piece of
equipment'. He feels that students are not interested in his experience of the
illness, but only in what they can get out of their interactions with him.

Victor also feels that students don't show any interest in what he is going
through, because they are only focused on the diagnosis. Having students listen
to your heart murmur can be a dehumanising experience for many people,
because it is often carried out without asking any questions and the patient is
asked not to speak because it interferes with hearing the sounds (Rice, 2008). If
a person's murmur is rare, they may be approached by large numbers of students
and junior doctors, all wanting to listen without engaging them in conversation.

This makes Victor feel that he is being treated 'like a dummy'. This term has
many connotations: it can refer to a mannequin, a person of low intelligence,
one who is unable to speak, or the subject of experimentation. He makes a plea
for an opportunity to share a little of his personal story with students; this, he
thinks, would be a fair exchange for the benefit they gain from being allowed to
examine him. Lynn Gillam's story about students carrying out an internal
examination at the instruction of a senior doctor, without her consent, highlights
the distress that can result from such everyday experiences of medical dehumanisation (Guillemin & Gillam, 2006).

The danger of conflating objectivity, an attitude that can be constructive in
medicine, with objectification is highlighted in Victor and Robin's stories. Being

used as a passive object for teaching can be an unpleasant experience. Treating patients as objects subject to manipulation is inconsistent with good medical practice, which should prioritise patients' needs and preferences (Australian Medical Council, 2014). Learning with and from patients instead of merely on or about them should minimise the risk of objectivity being confused or conflated with objectification (Bleakley & Bligh, 2008).

The patient as adversary

Stories told by Grace and Natalie about ward rounds and procedures show that, in some contexts, students identify doctors as allies while patients are identified as adversaries whose interests conflict with those of the students. When he talks about recruiting patients for tutorials, Robert implies that some degree of coercion may be justified close to exams or when patients have rare signs. He claims that patients shouldn't say 'no' to seeing students unless they are very unwell or distressed. Grace tells about her experiences asking patients if she can carry out procedures on them, and actually performing them. She admits that the process they have been taught to follow to ensure valid consent is often disregarded when students are trying to get opportunities to practice procedures.

Grace's narrative performance suggests ambivalence towards ethically suspect practices, but she attempts to justify subtle degrees of coercion from doctors and the concealment of students' status. She portrays patients' interests as being opposed to those of students, and as a result they sometimes appear as adversaries, who could thwart students' need for practical experience. Although she acknowledges that having an inexperienced student carry out a procedure can result in additional pain or distress, she fails to affirm the need for free and fully informed consent. Through her storytelling, Grace demonstrates that she complies with some expectations from her teachers in relation to practising procedures, for example by concealing her student status. However, she resists other expectations, when she declines to attempt a procedure without a supervisor, or more than once if unsuccessful. In this way she highlights her own agency and plays an active part in her identity construction.

Natalie's story focuses on an incident during a ward round, when students were asked to leave by the patient who was being seen by a doctor. The story explores her perceptions of customary practices of informing patients and obtaining their consent. Natalie was shocked when the patient insisted on them leaving, despite the doctor's efforts to advocate for the students. Natalie constructs the patient as an adversary and the doctor as the students' ally, claiming the patient was unreasonable despite having the right to decline to see students. She admits that on ward rounds, students are not often introduced as such. Natalie justifies this practice on the grounds that if patients *were* informed, they would refuse, and students would not get enough experience observing doctors at work.

Another student, named Thao, confides that he is concerned about how he will cope with repeated encounters with distressed patients, and disillusioned about the apparent cynicism he observes amongst many members of the profession he aspires to join. Thao is asked by a surgeon to examine a patient's breast without her consent, after telling her she probably has a recurrence of her cancer. He feels uncomfortable about being there, let alone conducting the examination, and shocked at the surgeon's apparent lack of concern for the patient's distress. In this story, Thao empathises and aligns himself with the patient, and portrays the doctor in a negative light, arguably as an adversary.

In a tutorial about challenging communication, Daniel emphasises the importance of considering how a patient's previous life experience might influence their feelings about having an intimate examination. He urges students to remember that they must always respect each patient's choice. His attitude contrasts with that of Robert, whose respect for patient choice is conditional on his opinion about the potential benefit for students or junior doctors.

Humanising clinical teaching

To move towards a dialogic medical education, students and their clinical teachers need to be aware that identity construction is one of the driving forces behind patients' storytelling in the context of clinical teaching. As I have shown, a person can identify themselves as a unique individual by telling stories about their life, and by having them heard and acknowledged. Although students and clinical teachers also do identity work through storytelling, the desire to do so can be especially critical for patients, who are often highly vulnerable and dependent on hospital staff. When people find themselves in an unfamiliar and impersonal location like a hospital ward, without personal clothing, possessions and other symbols of their identity, this can intensify their desire to identify themselves in relation to those around them, through storytelling (Monrouxe, Rees, & Bradley, 2009).

Consistent with the findings of other scholars, many of the patient stories in this book describe experiences of dehumanisation or objectification associated with their participation in medical students' learning (Monrouxe et al., 2009; Rice, 2008). Examples include the stories of Victor and Robin, who felt used or exploited, like a piece of equipment or a dummy. Although the three accounts of the tutorial with Brian highlight different aspects of the interaction, all of them reveal moments in which his humanity was denied. A transformation in Brian's demeanour was evident when his stories were repeatedly shut down and when he was spoken about in a demeaning way. Along with the findings from prior research, these accounts of circumstances in which people have experienced objectification during clinical teaching point to opportunities to humanise clinical teaching practice (Rees, Ajjawi, & Monrouxe, 2013). Some of these have already been described or advocated in stories in this book from clinical teachers like Daniel, Veronica and William.

Social psychology research into the ways people identify with social groups offers insight into the different ways in which students can identify with the medical profession (Roccas, Sagiv, Schwartz, Halevy, & Eidelson, 2008). If a student's mode of identification with the profession is predominantly through glorification (encompassing superiority and deference), they will be less willing to constructively criticise members of that group if they act in ways inconsistent with the group's stated aims. This might be a factor when students observe doctors disregarding proper consent procedures. On the other hand, if a student identifies predominantly through attachment (encompassing the importance of the group and how much they want to benefit it), they may be willing to con-structively criticise members of the group if they contravene its stated values.

Engaging dialogically

Another important requirement for a dialogic medical education is to recognise what it means to engage dialogically with another person. This is related to the idea of empathy because it requires a person to imagine the experiences and per-spective of the person they are interacting with, while continuing to be aware of their own separateness. Bakhtin argued that human existence or *being* – analogous to identity – is an ongoing *event*, which is always shared with others (Holquist, 2002). From this perspective, individual subjects can only know themselves in relation to other people; this is relevant to clinical communication and the ways in which knowledge and understanding emerge from it.

In his meditation on generosity in health care, Arthur Frank argues that ethical human interaction requires us to respect the *alterity* of others with whom we interact: their essential *otherness* (Frank, 2004). When a doctor interprets a patient's actions or motivation only from their own perspective, they fail to respect that patient's alterity. This can signal to a patient that their past experience is considered irrelevant to their healing, and the history and values informing their choices will be disregarded. Another potential consequence of failing to respect the other's alterity is the over-identification of the doctor with their patient. This is not in the patient's interest either, because it denies them the benefit of the doc-tor's knowledge and professional judgement. Meaningful dialogue in the context of health care interactions requires both the patient's and the doctor's perspectives – and often those of others, such as parents or care providers – to build a compre-hensive account of the patient's problems and potential remedies.

I have explored in a previous paper the idea of *practising engagement* as a way to engage in a dialogic clinical encounter (Warmington, 2012). I described engagement in this context as being made up of three actions: *attentiveness*, *authentic dialogue* and *commitment*, and offered a fictionalised account of a clin-ical encounter to show how they can be put into effect in everyday practice. If I engage dialogically with another person, I recognise that they cannot be *final-ised*; I am open to new insights into their situation and understanding of them as a person. However, if I engage with that person monologically, I interpret their actions only from my own perspective, considering myself qualified to have the last word, or to finalise them. As I write about the storytellers in this book and their characters, I strive to engage with them dialogically, and avoid claiming to have the last word on who they are. Examples of both ways of engaging with people can be found in many of the stories in this book, a selection of which is shown below.

Opportunities for dialogic transformation

I am arguing for the universal adoption of practices that promote dialogic engagement between students, clinical teachers and patients. The development and introduction of such practices must be tailored for local cultures and conditions, if they are to be accepted and sustained. A number of opportunities for change have emerged from this study, and others have been recommended by researchers in the published literature. Some of these would already be in

MONOLOGIC ENGAGEMENT: FINALISED	DIALOGIC ENGAGEMENT: UNFINALISED
	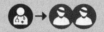
NATALIE (student about a patient):	**ASHANKA** (student about patients):
A patient said no on a ward round, and said: "Who **are** all these people? I don't want them here!" I'd **never** seen a patient exercise the right before to demand that we leave. We were pretty disappointed at that.	My tutor said, "You need to learn how to cut them off!" But I don't know **how** to cut them off, because they have to **tell** me things and to **them** it's important! I know, to the **history** it's not, but to them it **is**!
	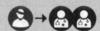
HARVEY (Patient about a student):	**HARVEY** (Patient about students):
It felt like he was trying to get a boost on all the other ones that were there. I just didn't want him trying to do a one-up-manship and using me to do that one-up-manship. I don't like people like that.	I've had some that I've thought they're not the right person to be a doctor. But I won't shoot **them** down. That's not up to me, it's up to their teachers, or they might talk to someone, click into it and do it right.
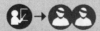	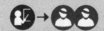
ROBERT (Clinical teacher about patients):	**DANIEL** (Clinical teacher about patients):
It's spelt out in the hospital brochures - "You may have medical students coming to talk to you. We encourage you to participate." So, I think that patients shouldn't really say no. I wouldn't say no.	In the end, don't forget that we have to respect their choice. You need to think about the person's cultural and personal background and how that might affect their feelings about the examination.

Figure 8.1 Monologic and dialogic engagement.

operation in some medical schools, but there is a need for them to be more widely implemented. I propose some changes, but this is not an exhaustive list, and readers will undoubtedly come up with their own, locally appropriate solutions. Firstly, I consider the clinical encounter itself, for example at the bedside or in the clinic, including any subsequent discussions. Secondly, I focus on the design and delivery of medical school curricula and, finally, I address the institutional and professional contexts in which medical education takes place.

Clinical teaching encounters

There is scope to involve patients in clinical teaching encounters more actively and respectfully, through awareness and discussion with students of some challenging issues. These include the potential for coercion or duplicity in the recruitment of patients, and the risk of dehumanisation and the silencing of patients' voices. In some situations, such as ward rounds, patients may not be asked if they agree to students being present or even informed that they are there. When students are learning and practising minor procedures on patients, they sometimes deliberately fail to disclose their status and inexperience. Consent should always be fully informed and free from coercion or duplicity.

When doctors are present, students often feel unable to intervene, even if they are concerned that a patient is unwilling or the interaction disrespectful, due to the power dynamics of the situation. Consequently, clinical teachers have a responsibility to ensure that patients who participate only do so if valid consent is obtained. They should also ensure they are adequately prepared, treated as active participants and have an opportunity to debrief afterwards. Given the vulnerable and dependent position of hospital patients, they should be explicitly told that they can decline to be involved or withdraw at any time without negative consequences. They should be informed what would be expected of them should they agree, including how many students will be involved, for how long, what they will be asked to do and whether there will be any opportunity to engage in conversation.

Certain types of encounters are inherently more objectifying, for example when students are asked to examine a patient without any preceding history or conversation. Clinical teachers could mitigate this risk by making time for some conversation before the examination, or if this is not possible, informing the patient of the potential for them to feel objectified as a result. Explicit reflection about the patient's involvement in a particular encounter could be incorporated into the teaching that takes place after the tutor and students have left them. Students could reflect on whether the patient shared personal stories and, if so, what they learnt from them and how this knowledge could be relevant to their medical care. They could discuss how the power dynamics of the interaction can inhibit those in subordinate positions from speaking up about their concerns, and how this could be addressed.

Addressing patients in a demeaning way or speaking about them as if they were not present is disrespectful and should be avoided. It is potentially harmful to their well-being and can also have consequences for students' identity construction. The use of jargon in front of patients can cause increased anxiety, so it should be avoided if possible or otherwise translated into plain language for the patient. During a short debriefing after every bedside teaching session, clinical teachers could clarify anything a patient has not understood with them, allay any concerns about what has been discussed and ask for feedback about their experience (Chretien, Goldman, Craven, & Faselis, 2010; Nair, Coughlan, & Hensley, 1997; Romano, 1941).

This study confirms that the clinical teaching encounter is a highly complex social interaction. As a result, it can be difficult for students and teachers to focus simultaneously on the technical aspects of a task and on the patient's comfort. One way to reduce the risk of patients having negative experiences would be for clinical teachers to ask one of the students to focus on the patient's well-being and to interrupt the session if the patient appears uncomfortable or in need of a break. They could also be asked to act as a timekeeper and interrupt the session if it is taking longer than expected, so the patient can be offered the option to finish if they have had enough.

Students could be invited to reflect on how their clinical teacher interacted with a patient, for example, how well they focused on the patient's needs and how the patient responded. Although many students would be reluctant to criticise their teacher because of their position of authority, this barrier could be overcome if they were encouraged to do so. As well as benefiting patients, these innovations could make students more aware of the embodied signs of patient discomfort and the need to prioritise patient interests, and help teachers improve the quality of their own interactions. They could foster a sense of empowerment, preparing students to speak up in future if they witness troubling interactions involving other clinicians.

During this study, many students and their teachers expressed the view that fully informed patients would not be willing to participate in students' education. They used this argument to support ethically dubious recruitment practices. However, many patients in this study, like those in prior research, gave a number of altruistic and self-interested reasons for their willingness to be involved (Chretien et al., 2010; Fletcher, Rankey, & Stern, 2005; McLachlan, King, Wenger, & Dornan, 2012). Therefore, it seems unlikely that seeking fully informed consent would result in students losing access to patients. In any case, hospital patients are not obliged to participate and should always make the choice to do so as freely as possible, even though consent is inherently complicated when people are recipients of care in the same institution (Waterbury, 2001).

One argument against many of the changes I and other researchers have suggested is that they would increase the time spent on each clinical interaction. This is a valid concern, because there is limited time available for clinical teaching, whether in formal tutorials or incidental to doctors' work. The number of patients seen by each student would probably be reduced if these strategies were implemented, but patients' active participation should be enhanced, and the risk of dehumanising experiences minimised. They should also have a positive effect on students' learning and the identities constructed during these interactions. I argue that the increased

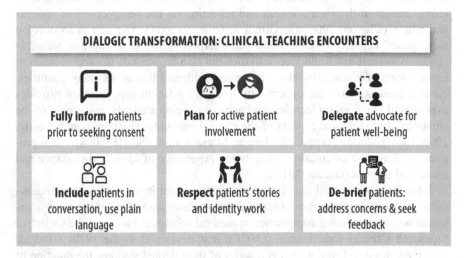

Figure 8.2 Dialogic transformation: clinical teaching encounters.

value in terms of the quality of the interactions and students' learning and identity would outweigh any disadvantages from the reduced number of patients seen.

Curriculum design and delivery

The kinds of changes I have suggested are linked to curriculum design, delivery and assessment and would require leadership and support from medical school faculty members. A crucial component would be enhanced training and support for clinical teachers. A formal supervision arrangement for their teaching role should also be considered, given their key influence on students' learning and identity formation. As part of their training, clinical teachers should learn about how identity construction takes place as an integral part of the acquisition of clinical knowledge and skills. The use of storytelling and reflective discussion, as employed in this book, can provide valuable insights into the links between identity, power and practice in clinical settings (Bleakley, Bligh, & Browne, 2011).

Academic medical educators should take into account the potential for emotional distress as a result of identity dissonance, which can arise when the attitudes and practices expected of a student's emerging professional identity conflict with those of their established identities (Goldie, 2012; Monrouxe, 2010). These experiences can have adverse effects on students' well-being and performance. Although medical schools offer psychological services and pastoral care to students, many students are reluctant to identify themselves as having a problem, fearing stigma or a negative impact on the school's assessment of their competence (Goldie, 2012; Monrouxe, 2010).

Medical schools can incorporate strategies to support students' identity construction, including guided reflective activities. One approach introduces narrative medicine by way of the *parallel chart*. This involves students or junior doctors telling stories of their experiences and reflecting on the perspectives of patients and others (Charon, 2006; DasGupta & Charon, 2004). The aim is to develop participants' capacity to understand and interpret stories in a way that enhances clinical relationships. Reflective activities can also incorporate the appreciation of literary texts or visual artworks relating to health and illness. In many countries, medical students have the opportunity to attend a Balint group, which provides experiential small group learning and aims to develop students' awareness of the emotional and relational aspects of the clinical encounter (Lichtenstein & Lustig, 2006; Lustig, 2008; Torppa, Makkonen, Mårtenson, & Pitkälä, 2008). Such programmes have the potential to mitigate the experience of identity dissonance and associated distress (Goldie, 2012).

It has been recognised that the nature of assessment in any educational endeavour is a powerful influence on what and how students learn. One of the most widespread ways of assessing competence in medical schools is known as the Objective Structured Clinical Examination (OSCE), first developed in the 1970s (Hodges, 2003). As discussed earlier, this is a series of time limited stations, the duration of which varies, but in Australia it is typically eight minutes. Many of these stations require students to gather information about a body system by interviewing a real or simulated patient or performing an examination. They may be designed to assess performance on other tasks, such as clinical communication. Examiners observe and assess each candidate's performance using highly structured scoring instruments.

This approach to assessment has become ubiquitous in the interest of standardisation, reliability and fairness for candidates. However, one consequence of this format may be a reduction in students' capacity to appreciate the subtleties of clinical interactions (Hodges, 2003). Although there has been considerable research examining the reliability and psychometric characteristics of the OSCE, there has been little investigation into its impact on medical training and practice (Hodges, 2003; Huntley, Salmon, Fisher, Fletcher, & Young, 2012). During their tutorials and individual practice with patients, students and their tutors are aware that they will need to perform particular routines of history-taking or examination of a body system in order to pass their exams. This can lead to a body system-centred form of learning, which does not prepare students well for the complexities of clinical practice.

Modifications to the standard structure of the OSCE have been proposed to address some of its perceived shortcomings. In Canada, the problem of fragmentation of complex clinical problems which occurs with isolated brief stations was addressed with a modified OSCE format (Hatala, Marr, Cuncic, & Bacchus, 2011). This required candidates to interact with a single standardised patient over three linked ten-minute stations, which addressed the physical examination, management and communication skills. Most candidates and examiners considered this to be more realistic and to overcome some of the limitations of the standard OSCE format (Hatala et al., 2011).

Since communication is an inherently creative endeavour, it has been argued that poor communication is more likely to reflect limitations in a candidate's knowledge, values or emotional processes than a lack of particular skills (Huntley et al., 2012). An instrument known as the Liverpool Undergraduate Communication Assessment Scale (LUCAS) enables faculty to assess how well the communication met the needs of the patient, not only whether the student displayed particular behaviour or skills (Huntley et al., 2012).

Simulated interactions have a place, for example to practice the sequence of tasks involved in a particular physical examination or a particular technical skill. However, I believe authentic patient encounters, supported by appropriate feedback, should form the basis for students' learning about clinical communication and relationships. As a result of early and extensive reliance on simulation-based learning, medical students may expect real patients to present their stories in a linear and coherent fashion. They may see a patient as a series of disconnected body systems and pay insufficient attention to their illness experience. These problems could be mitigated if genuine patients were engaged in the design of simulated scenarios. There is scope for more patient participation in curriculum design more broadly; in one study, a problem-based learning case was based on the first-hand experiences of a patient with a psychiatric illness (Chur-Hansen & Koopowitz, 2004). Students could also be encouraged to reflect on the *differences* between authentic and simulated interactions.

In this study, I have shown that some patients evaluate students on the basis of their behaviour. Sometimes, they empathise with students' perceived emotional discomfort and form judgements about their character. There is potential for patients' evaluations of their interactions with students to be used more widely as a resource to support students' learning. They could be incorporated into the process of debriefing, which should be undertaken after every clinical teaching interaction, in a similar way to the participation of trained teaching associates to train students how to perform sensitive examinations appropriately (Robertson, Hegarty, O'Connor, &

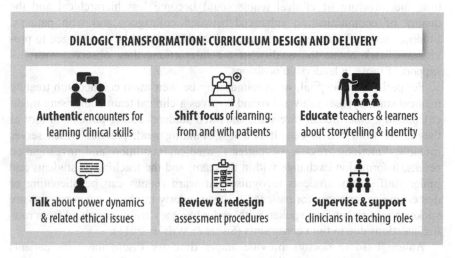

DIALOGIC TRANSFORMATION: CURRICULUM DESIGN AND DELIVERY

Authentic encounters for learning clinical skills

Shift focus of learning: from and with patients

Educate teachers & learners about storytelling & identity

Talk about power dynamics & related ethical issues

Review & redesign assessment procedures

Supervise & support clinicians in teaching roles

Figure 8.3 Dialogic transformation: curriculum design and delivery.

Gunn, 2003; Hendrickx et al., 2006). Some patients may be reluctant to express negative views in front of students, so written feedback could be an option.

Students also learn from clinicians whose interactions they observe during workplace activities such as ward rounds or clinics; this is an example of situated learning (Lave & Wenger, 1991). The ways in which these doctors relate to patients can have profound effects on the students' emerging professional identities. I address the challenge involved in changing the attitudes, values and practices of clinicians who have a strong influence on students' tacit learning in the next section.

Institutional and professional cultures

Both the profession of medicine and the institution of the hospital have their own cultures: accumulations of shared values, practices and objectives. Their influences on students' identity formation extend well beyond the clinical school and staff engaged in formal teaching. The culture of medicine has been characterised as strongly individualistic, presenting a façade of invulnerability and a denial of personal susceptibility to illness or stress (Kirschbaum & Fortner, 2012). In a teaching hospital, medical students tacitly learn what is expected of them as they observe doctors in their everyday practice. Although they are inspired and encouraged by many of the interactions they witness, they find others ethically troubling, but may feel unable to speak up about them due to strong constraints against criticising those in superior positions.

Parallels have been drawn between aspects of medical teamwork and those in other occupations where safety and risk management are crucial, such as the aviation industry. This has highlighted the importance of human factors such as leadership, communication and occupational culture in avoiding critical incidents or 'near miss' events and responding to them when they do occur (Schenkel, 2000). If this way of thinking were applied to clinical communication, the structure of clinical teams could become less hierarchical and the quality of communication enhanced between colleagues and with patients. Students and staff, as well as patients and families, could be encouraged to provide feedback about the quality of the interactions they observe, with full support of those in leadership positions.

For patients in hospital, ward rounds may be their main contact with treating medical staff. Typically, a ward round involves a clinical team comprising medical, nursing, other health care staff, and often students seeing patients in turn as they move from bed to bed. It is a long-standing work practice which serves multiple functions: review of patients' medical condition and investigation results, information exchange within the team, and the teaching of students and junior staff. Many students recognise that ward rounds can be alienating or demeaning experiences for patients. It is particularly troubling when patients are spoken about rather than spoken with, and when they are discouraged from raising questions due to time constraints (Sweet & Wilson, 2011).

Although some doctors provide ample time for discussion with patients during rounds, others typically see a large number of patients in a short time, which can result in patients lacking an opportunity to speak and feeling that their concerns have not been addressed. Although ward rounds are considered an efficient use of staff time, there is scope to consider changes to the structure of ward rounds to ensure that they address patients' needs as well as those of staff.

The 'Family-Centered Bedside Round' was developed as a new way of conducting ward rounds for clinical care and teaching in an acute paediatric unit (Muething, Kotagal, Shoettker, Gonzalez del Rey, & De Witt, 2007). This was a response to a policy statement from the American Academy of Pediatrics and the Institute for Family-Centered Care, requiring clinicians to actively involve families at the hospital bedside. Most families chose to be involved and there was a strong emphasis on introducing team members, facilitating parents' contributions to discussions and respecting them as the experts on their own child. Despite some staff members' initial concerns, it was eventually accepted enthusiastically by most of those involved. It is valued as an opportunity for students and junior staff to learn respect for the concerns of patients and families and develop their capacity to build collaborative relationships with them (Muething et al., 2007).

One of the inevitable tensions in clinical work, and particularly hospital ward rounds, relates to time management: the need for sufficient time to be allocated to each patient for their medical condition and concerns to be adequately addressed, while enabling clinicians to complete all necessary tasks in the time available. One study compared the effects on patient perceptions of ward round interactions, when the doctor sat down at the bedside or stood beside it (Swayden et al., 2012). When doctors sat down, patients thought they had spent longer interacting with them, even though the actual time spent did not change significantly. Patients also felt they understood their condition better and were more satisfied with the interaction when their doctor sat down beside them. Increased patient satisfaction has been shown to enhance adherence to treatment advice, reduce the length of stay in hospital and improve clinical outcomes (Swayden et al., 2012). Relatively simple changes to the way clinicians interact with patients on ward rounds, such as sitting down beside them where possible, can have meaningful positive results for patient care.

There are inherent problems with ward rounds as currently structured in relation to practices of disclosure and consent. When students attend ward rounds, it is common for them not to be introduced as students, and patients may not be asked for permission to have them present. Potential reasons for this include a desire to maximise students' access to patients, time constraints and a lack of respect for patients' right to the privacy of their health-related information. Similar considerations apply when students wish to perform a procedure on a patient. Doctors may exert subtle pressure on patients to allow students to practise on them or fail to offer them the option of having a more experienced person. Medical students' attitudes towards telling patients that they are students tend to decline as they advance through medical school, but patients attach high importance to being informed (Silver-Isenstadt & Ubel, 1999).

Some of these practices need to be changed to promote positive identity development and guard against the erosion of ethical standards during medical training. There is the potential for changes to be implemented, even to long-standing practices (Muething et al., 2007). Such innovations could enhance students' future dealings with patients by promoting transparency, collaboration and mutual trust, which are essential for a healthy therapeutic relationship.

The rules governing the structure of the medical record and the clinical case presentation have a profound influence on clinical interactions. They shape the story that students or junior doctors construct, and therefore the nature of their interactions with patients (Donnelly, 1997, 2005; Holmes & Ponte, 2011). Therefore, a genuinely patient-centred medical record would be an essential element of dialogic medical education and care (Donnelly, 2005, p. 33). Incorporating questions about the patient's major concerns at each review is a small adjustment that could re-orient the tasks of history-taking and recording towards the patient's story.

My case in favour of a dialogic medical education is supported by the findings of my own research into the student-patient encounter, and by the work of others in this field. By integrating ethnography with dialogic narrative analysis, my research has brought to light new knowledge, including patients' experiences of empathy for students, and their judgements about students' character. My findings have also provided empirical support to other authors who have written about identity construction (Barr, Bull, & Rooney, 2015; Bleakley, Bligh, & Browne, 2011; Dornan, Pearson, Carson, Helmich, & Bundy, 2015; Gaufberg, Batalden, Sands, & Bell, 2010; Goldie, 2012; Monrouxe, 2010; Monrouxe & Poole, 2013; Schrewe, Bates, Pratt, Ruitenberg, & McKellin, 2017; Wortham, 2006), and those who have expressed concerns about the unintended consequences of learning by simulation and argued for more patient-centred clinical teaching (Bleakley & Bligh, 2008; Bligh & Bleakley, 2006).

This study opens the way for future research, including the study of relational identity construction in a variety of learning contexts, such as primary care and

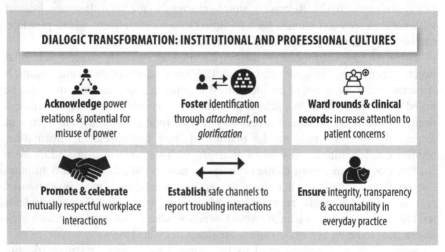

Figure 8.4 Dialogic transformation: institutional and professional cultures.

community settings, including those in rural and regional areas. Identity construction could be studied in simulated encounters and in reflective groups where people talk about their clinical interactions, such as narrative medicine groups and Balint groups (Charon, 2006; Torppa et al., 2008). Since identity construction is a dynamic and ongoing process, it would be valuable to study its emergence during formal postgraduate training programmes, or as a part of trainees' adaptation to new workplaces and contexts. A further research direction could be to investigate the impacts of established work practices and social structures at the institutional level, or political and economic constraints at the societal level, on students' identity formation.

Some of the stories in this book are ethically troubling, because they reveal how respect for the human rights of patients can be disregarded to serve the interests of staff or students. In recent years, a number of trusted institutions have been shown to have abrogated their responsibilities towards the people they were supposed to serve and protect. Examples include the commission and concealment of child sexual abuse within churches and state care homes, dishonest practices by financial institutions and the abuse and neglect of people living with disabilities. While the severity of harm in those cases far exceeds the effects on patients of the practices described in this book, there are some parallels. Patients in hospital are vulnerable and dependent on medical and other staff. Although they are often willing to help with students' learning, they should always have the choice whether to participate or not, and be fully informed as to what that would involve. Some of the practices routinely described by students and clinical teachers to recruit patients could be used to manipulate or deceive them. Such practices can result in patients feeling used or exploited and fail to meet the standards of honesty and respect expected of the profession.

Understanding how identity is constructed in everyday clinical encounters has the potential to enhance the well-being of medical students, doctors and their patients. By offering insights into how identities are constructed relationally in the context of medical education, this book makes the case for focusing on the identity work done by *patients*, alongside that of students and clinical teachers. The exploration of patients' identity formation has contributed original knowledge about the relational nature of identity. A move towards a dialogic medical education could positively transform clinical teaching encounters. It could enable them to be more collaborative and mutually satisfying and should promote more effective and rewarding relationships between doctors and their patients in contexts of clinical care.

References

Australian Medical Council. (2014). *Good medical practice – a code of conduct for doctors in Australia* (pp. 1–25). Medical Board of Australia. Retrieved from: www.medicalboard.gov.au/Codes-Guidelines-Policies/Code-of-conduct.aspx

Bakhtin, M. M. (1981). *The dialogic imagination: Four essays* (M. Holquist Ed.). Austin, TX: University of Texas Press.

Bakhtin, M. M. (1986). The problem of speech genres (V. W. McGee, Trans.). In C. Emerson & M. Holquist (Eds.), *Speech genres and other late essays* (pp. 60–102). Austin, TX: University of Texas Press.

Barr, J., Bull, R., & Rooney, K. (2015). Developing a patient focussed professional identity: An exploratory investigation of medical students' encounters with patient partnership in learning. *Advances in Health Sciences Education, 20*(2), 325–338. doi:10.1007/s10459-014-9530-8

Bleakley, A., & Bligh, J. (2008). Students learning from patients: Let's get real in medical education. *Advances in Health Sciences Education, 13*, 89–107.

Bleakley, A., Bligh, J., & Browne, J. (2011). *Medical education for the future: Identity, power and location*. London: Springer.

Bligh, J., & Bleakley, A. (2006). Distributing menus to hungry learners: Can learning by simulation become simulation of learning? *Medical Teacher, 28*(7), 606–613. doi:10.1080/01421590601042335

Charon, R. (2006). Chapter 8: The Parallel Chart. In *Narrative medicine: Honoring the stories of illness* (pp. 155–174). New York: Oxford University Press.

Chretien, K., Goldman, E., Craven, K., & Faselis, C. (2010). A qualitative study of the meaning of physical examination teaching for patients. *Journal of General Internal Medicine, 25*(8), 786–791.

Chur-Hansen, A., & Koopowitz, L. (2004). The patient's voice in a problem-based learning case. *Australasian Psychiatry, 12*(1), 31–35.

DasGupta, S., & Charon, R. (2004). Personal illness narratives: Using reflective writing to teach empathy. *Academic Medicine, 79*(4), 351–356.

Donnelly, W. J. (1997). The language of medical case histories. *Annals of Internal Medicine, 127*(11), 1045–1048.

Donnelly, W. J. (2005). Patient-centred medical care requires a patient-centred medical record. *Academic Medicine, 80*(1), 33–38.

Dornan, T., Pearson, E., Carson, P., Helmich, E., & Bundy, C. (2015). Emotions and identity in the figured world of becoming a doctor. *Medical Education, 49*, 174–185. doi:10.1111/medu12587

Fletcher, K., Rankey, D., & Stern, D. (2005). Bedside interactions from the other side of the bedrail. *Journal of General Internal Medicine, 20*, 58–61.

Frank, A. W. (2004). *The renewal of generosity: Illness, medicine and how to live*. Chicago, IL: The University of Chicago Press.

Gaufberg, E., Batalden, M., Sands, R., & Bell, S. (2010). The hidden curriculum: What can we learn from third-year medical student narrative reflections? *Academic Medicine, 85*, 1709–1716.

Goldie, J. (2012). The formation of professional identity in medical students: Considerations for educators. *Medical Teacher, 34*, e641–e648.

Guillemin, M., & Gillam, L. (2006). *Telling moments: Everyday ethics in health care*. Melbourne: IP Communications.

Hatala, R., Marr, S., Cuncic, C., & Bacchus, C. M. (2011). Modification of an OSCE format to enhance patient continuity in a high-stakes assessment of clinical performance. *BMC Medical Education, 11*(23), 1–5.

Hendrickx, K., De Winter, B. Y., Wyndaele, J.-J., Tjalma, W. A. A., Debaene, L., Selleslags, B., … Bossaert, L. (2006). Intimate examination teaching with volunteers: Implementation and assessment at the University of Antwerp. *Patient Education and Counseling, 63*(1–2), 47–54.

Hodges, B. (2003). OSCE! Variations on a theme by Harden. *Medical Education, 37,* 1134–1140.

Holmes, S., & Ponte, M. (2011). En-case-ing the patient: Disciplining uncertainty in medical student patient presentations. *Culture, Medicine and Psychiatry, 35,* 163–182. doi:10.1007/s11013-011-9213-3

Holquist, M. (2002). *Dialogism* (2nd ed.). London & New York: Routledge.

Huntley, C., Salmon, P., Fisher, P., Fletcher, I., & Young, B. (2012). LUCAS: A theoretically informed instrument to assess clinical communication in objective structured clinical examinations *Medical Education, 46,* 267–276. doi:10.1111/j.1365-2923. 2011.04162.x

Kirschbaum, K., & Fortner, S. (2012). Medical culture and communication. *Journal of Communication in Healthcare, 5*(3), 182–189. doi:10.1179/1753807612Y.0000000010

Lave, J., & Wenger, E. (1991). *Situated learning: Legitimate peripheral participation.* Cambridge: Cambridge University Press.

Lichtenstein, A., & Lustig, M. (2006). Integrating intuition and reasoning: How Balint groups can help medical decision making. *Australian Family Physician, 35*(12), 987–989.

Lustig, M. (2008). Letter: Humanising medical practice: The role of empathy. *Medical Journal of Australia, 188*(4), 263–264.

McLachlan, E., King, N., Wenger, E., & Dornan, T. (2012). Phenomenological analysis of patient experiences of medical student teaching encounters. *Medical Education, 46*(10), 963–973. doi:10.1111/j.1365-2923.2012.04332.x

Monrouxe, L. (2010). Identity, identification and medical education: Why should we care? *Medical Education, 44*(1), 40–49. doi:10.1111/j.1365-2923.2009.03440.x

Monrouxe, L., & Poole, G. (2013). An onion? Conceptualising and researching identity. *Medical Education, 47*(4), 425–429. doi:10.1111/medu.12123

Monrouxe, L., Rees, C., & Bradley, P. (2009). The construction of patients' involvement in hospital bedside teaching encounters. *Qualitative Health Research, 19*(7), 918–930. doi:10.1177/1049732309338583

Muething, S., Kotagal, U., Shoettker, P., Gonzalez del Rey, J., & De Witt, T. (2007). Family centered bedside rounds: A new approach to patient care and teaching. *Pediatrics, 119*(4), 829–832. doi: 10.1542/peds.2006-2528

Nair, B. R., Coughlan, J. L., & Hensley, M. J. (1997). Student and patient perspectives on bedside teaching. *Medical Education, 31,* 341–346.

Rees, C., Ajjawi, R., & Monrouxe, L. V. (2013). The construction of power in family medicine bedside teaching: A video observation study. *Medical Education, 47*(2), 154–165. doi:10.1111/medu.12055

Rice, T. (2008). 'Beautiful murmurs': Stethoscopic listening and acoustic objectification. *The Senses and Society, 3,* 293–306. doi:10.2752/174589308X331332

Robertson, K., Hegarty, K., O'Connor, V., & Gunn, J. (2003). Women teaching women's health: Issues in the establishment of a clinical teaching associate program for the well woman check. *Women & Health, 37*(4), 49–65. doi:10.1300/J013v37n04_05

Roccas, S., Sagiv, L., Schwartz, S., Halevy, N., & Eidelson, R. (2008). Toward a unifying model of identification with groups: Integrating theoretical perspectives. *Personality and Social Psychology Review, 12*(3), 280–306. doi:10.1177/1088868308319225

Romano, J. (1941). Patients' attitudes and behavior in ward round teaching. *JAMA (Chicago, Ill.), 117*(9), 664–667.

Schenkel, S. (2000). Promoting patient safety and preventing medical error in emergency departments. *Academic Emergency Medicine, 7*(11), 1204–1222. doi:10.1111/ j.1553-2712.2000.tb00466.x

Schrewe, B., Bates, J., Pratt, D., Ruitenberg, C. W., & McKellin, W. H. (2017). The Big D(eal): Professional identity through discursive constructions of 'patient'. *Medical Education, 51*(6), 656–668. doi:10.1111/medu.13299

Silver-Isenstadt, A., & Ubel, P. A. (1999). Erosion in medical students' attitudes about telling patients they are students. *Journal of General Internal Medicine, 14*(8), 481–487.

Swayden, K., Anderson, K., Connelly, L., Moran, J., McMahon, J., & Arnold, P. (2012). Effect of sitting vs. standing on perception of provider time at bedside: A pilot study. *Patient Education and Counselling, 87*(2), 166–171. doi:10.1016/j.pec.2011.05.024

Sweet, G. S., & Wilson, H. J. (2011). A patient's experience of ward rounds. *Patient Education and Counselling, 84*(2), 150–151. doi:10.1016/j.pec.2010.08.016

Torppa, M., Makkonen, E., Mårtenson, C., & Pitkälä, K. (2008). A qualitative analysis of student Balint groups in medical education: Contexts and triggers of case presentations and discussion themes. *Patient Education and Counselling, 72*, 5–11.

Vågan, A. (2011). Towards a sociocultural perspective on identity formation in education. *Mind, Culture, and Activity, 18*(1), 43–57. doi:10.1080/10749031003605839

Warmington, S. (2012). Practising engagement: Infusing communication with empathy and compassion within medical students' clinical encounters. *Health: An Interdisciplinary Journal for the Study of Health, Illness and Medicine, 16*(3), 324–339. doi: 10.1177/1363459311416834

Waterbury, J. T. (2001). Refuting patients' obligations to clinical training: A critical analysis of the arguments for an obligation of patients to participate in the clinical education of medical students. *Medical Education, 35*(3), 286–294.

Wortham, S. (2000). Interactional positioning and narrative self-construction. *Narrative Inquiry, 10*(1), 157–184. doi:10.1075/ni.10.1.11wor

Wortham, S. (2006). *Learning identity: The joint emergence of social identification and academic learning.* New York: Cambridge University Press.

Index

Page numbers in *italics* denote figures

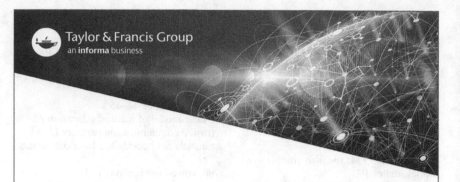

Printed in the United States
by Baker & Taylor Publisher Services